Emergency Medical Care: The Neglected Public Service

Emergency Medical Care: The Neglected Public Service

The Connecticut Experience

Alfred M. Sadler, Jr., M.D.
Blair L. Sadler, J.D.
Samuel B. Webb, Jr., Dr.P.H.

Ballinger Publishing Company • Cambridge, Massachusetts
A Subsidiary of J.B. Lippincott Company

International Standard Book Number: 0-88410-126-6

Library of Congress Catalog Card Number: 76-27275

Printed in the United States of America

Library of Congress Cataloging in Publication Data

Sadler, Alfred Mitchell, 1941–
   Emergency medical care.

   Includes bibliographical references.
   1. Emergency medical services—Connecticut. I. Sadler, Blair L., joint author.
II. Webb, Samuel B., joint author. III. Title.
RA645.6.C8S2   362.1   76-27275
ISBN 0-88410-126-6

To Dr. Jack W. Cole who, as chairman of the Yale University School of Medicine's Department of Surgery, opened up important avenues of thought and resources to us. His inspiration, leadership, and friendship were invaluable.

Summary of Contents

Part IV
Improving the System

Contents

List of Figures

xv

List of Tables

Foreword

In 1970, when this study began, emergency medical care was a neglected public service. This was true in Connecticut and indeed in most of the country. That it is less neglected now is due in large part to this and similar studies. The questions asked in the various chapters of the book were either answered or labeled as unanswerable in light of present documented experience. In either case the need for reliable information or change was well documented. In this sense, the book is an example of good journalism as well as good research—the proper questions were directed toward decision-makers and with broad public interests in mind.

The recommendations as to what to do, who should do it, priority setting, and time framework are particular for the State of Connecticut during the study period of 1970–73. The process, however, is nearly universal in terms of what questions to ask, to whom to direct them, essential social components, and conclusions drawn. In this sense, the importance of the book is in its methodology and its "blueprint for change."

It is impressive that just three years after the completion of the study, nearly all of the recommendations made have been adopted. This is probably not coincidental since considerable attention was given by the study team to the appropriate mechanisms for implementing these recommendations. Although the book makes no attempt to analyze in detail the actual process of implementation, the approach described offers important insights about transforming recommendations into implementation.

Unfortunately, the neglect mentioned in the book's title is still all too true in many areas of the country where emergency care remains undefined in terms of need and unresolved in terms of direction. This book should be valuable to the many planners, physicians, and policy-makers around the country who are becomming committed to improved emergency medical care.

Eugene L. Nagel, M.D.
Anesthesiologist-in-Chief
The Johns Hopkins Hospital
Baltimore, Maryland

Preface

Anyone who has attempted to study and improve emergency medical services has undoubtedly been humbled by the experience. Emergency medical crises are both unpredictable in their occurrence and complex in their management—involving as they do a wide variety of medical disciplines, a mixture of public and private resources (including police, fire, and ambulance services), a diversity of hospitals, and often multijurisdictional arrangements. Indeed, there are so many components that could be improved if quality emergency medical care were to be available to everyone, changes in most parts of emergency medical systems are sufficiently difficult and slow to implement, and the ability to measure the impact of such changes so limited, that this field is hardly one for those who look for quick, short-term solutions.

It is all the more humbling to those involved in improving emergency medical services (EMS) when some external factor, such as the reduction of highway speed limits (a reduction caused primarily by the gasoline shortage, rather than by a carefully planned decision by health care providers, consumers, or their elected representatives), may have saved as many lives in the past few years as any single change in the actual delivery of emergency care.

Programs to educate the public in safer driving or in the early warning signs of heart attacks, legislation requiring mandatory inclusion of seat belts in all new automobiles or more strict drunken driving standards, and efforts to train the public in cardiopulmonary resuscitation techniques all have their strong advocates. Whatever the success of these programs, however, they will never eliminate the need to improve the nation's capacity to respond to medical emergencies once they occur. Effective emergency care systems will always be necessary.

Improvements in emergency medical services in Connecticut received a boost in 1967 when, upon returning from active service in Vietnam, Dr. Kristaps J. Keggi, formerly assistant professor of orthopedic surgery at the Yale University School of Medicine, received a $30,000 grant from the Travellers Research Center in Hartford, Connecticut, to study trauma from a multidisciplinary perspective. Subsequently Dr. Jack W. Cole, chairman of the Department of Surgery at Yale, set out to establish a firm base from which to conduct vitally needed multidisciplinary research and education, and to act as a catalyst for reform. In 1969, Dr. Cole sought the support of the Commonwealth Fund of New York to establish the Yale Trauma Program.

In the proposal to the Commonwealth Fund, Dr. Cole noted:

> Although most schools have devoted a great deal of time toward achieving a better understanding of the biological, physiological, and biochemical derangements of the human organism resulting from trauma, insufficient effort and research have gone into ... the psychological, sociological, medicolegal, rehabilitative, and transportation fields. In short, to the best of our knowledge, no medical school has seen fit to embrace ... all of the areas that bear on the health care system dealing with the post-accident phase of injury. To develop such a broadly-based, multidisciplinary unit under the aegis of a leading medical school would indeed be unique, and its capacity to enlist the help and cooperation of responsible groups in government, industry and the lay community should eventuate in model systems for the care of the trauma victim."[1]

The report also noted that significant research in accidents and emergency care problems had already been conducted at Yale by Dr. Jerome Beloff, Professor Guido Calabresi, Dr. William Collins, Dr. Kristaps Keggi, Professor John Thompson, Dr. Samuel Webb, the late Dr. Richard Weinerman, and others. The award of a substantial grant from the Commonwealth Fund in December 1969 formally launched the Yale Trauma Program. In 1970, Dr. Alfred Sadler and Mr. Blair Sadler left the National Institutes of Health to assume the leadership of the Trauma Program.

In 1970, Connecticut was not a leader in emergency medical services. There was little knowledge of existing resources statewide, a paucity of even minimum standards and no mechanism for bringing the many relevant groups involved together. Thus, one of the first efforts of the Yale Trauma Program was to undertake a comprehensive study of EMS strengths and deficiencies in Connecticut.

This book is a detailed collaborative account of the way we went about this effort, the lessons we learned, the things we observed, the recommendations we made, the priorities we developed, the strategy we set, and the timetable we established. The final chapter presents a brief account of events since the submission of the study to Governor Thomas Meskill on December 15, 1972.

Probably the most striking study finding is the small investment of public funds in emergency ambulance services when compared with police and fire services. Our estimated cost of quality emergency ambulance service is approximately $2.00 per person per year. We view emergency ambulance care as a third public emergency service deserving comparable attention and public support.

We are pleased that in the past three and one-half years, most of the recommendations made have been implemented, including the enactment of strong enabling legislation at the state level. EMS is emerging as a priority health activity in Connecticut. While we take little credit for these recent developments, we do believe that the study and its recommendations set the stage for the changes that have occurred and are continuing to occur.

Many individuals contributed to this effort. Thomas Brask and Carol von Stein of the Yale Trauma Program were heavily involved in the planning and data analysis phases. Karen Bratsenis and Dr. Richard Pepler of Dunlap and Associates contributed to the data analysis and provided important consultation and critical review.

The staff and faculty of the Yale-New Haven Hospital and the Yale Medical School were most cooperative. Particularly helpful were Dr. Courtney Bishop, formerly chief of staff at Yale-New Haven Hospital; Ann Bliss and Paul Moson, Yale Trauma Program; Dr. Thomas Krizek, professor of surgery; Dr. Lawrence Pickett, professor of surgery and chief of staff, Yale-New Haven Hospital; Paul Lally, coordinator of emergency services, Yale-New Haven Hospital; and Charles Womer, president, Yale-New Haven Hospital.

Nine former students of the Master's Program in Hospital Administration at Yale Medical School's Department of Epidemiology and Public Health labored with us in designing the study, collecting much of the basic data and assisting in initial data analysis. They are Stephen Beloff, Paul Bushnell, John Drew, Henry Fenhagen, Eugene Richardson, Gerald Starr, Kent Stevens, Fred Vago, and John Weber.

Judith Castellon, Mary Beth Graham, and Linda Parkes painstakingly retyped many drafts of the original report submitted to Governor Meskill. Merle Spiegel's editorial assistance and Diane Montagne's secretarial assistance were invaluable in preparing the manuscript for publication.

The assistance of the original Connecticut Advisory Committee on Emergency Medical Services was vital. While we did not all agree on every issue, the interchange and discussion was always open, candid, and lively. (The members of the Advisory Committee are listed in Appendix 2A.)

We are particularly grateful to Robert Bergeron, who provided an institutional home for committee meetings at the Connecticut Hospital Association, as well as valuable advice and counsel. Finally, we are pleased to acknowledge the Commonwealth Fund of New York, particularly Quigg Newton and Terrance Keenan, whose generous support made this effort possible.

A.M.S., Jr.
B.L.S.
S.B.W., Jr.

Boston, Massachusetts
Princeton, New Jersey
New Haven, Connecticut
November, 1976

✳ *Part I*

Perspective and Planning

Chapter 1

EMS in Perspective: The Past Decade

Emergency medical services (EMS) is one of the most widely discussed health topics in the United States today.

This is not surprising since heart attacks and accidents are two of the country's major killers and it is widely believed that prompt quality emergency medical care could save many lives and reduce the severity of many injuries.

And yet, as recently as ten years ago, EMS was a neglected area of health care. Many ambulance services were run by funeral homes and most services were staffed by inadequately trained personnel. Hospital emergency rooms were often understaffed and poorly organized.

More fundamentally, in most parts of the country, no one had assumed clear-cut responsibility for EMS. Unlike police and fire services with high visibility, strong national organizations, and a position of prominence at state and local levels, ambulance services were often neglected and ignored. Unlike the development of sophisticated techniques and systems of managing certain specialized health care problems, emergency medicine was not given a priority by the nation's medical schools. Little research was being done and many young Americans were receiving an M.D. degree without having been taught the basics of emergency medicine. Small wonder then that many physicians felt ill equipped to respond to emergencies in such common instances as the roadside accident.

Although the country awoke to these problems in the late 1960s, Dr. Edgar Lee was certainly correct when, in 1970, he stated at an International Trauma Symposium that:

The study and treatment of trauma are not just neglected; in many instances they are actively suppressed. For too many years too many people have considered it such an undignified, untidy, and heterogeneous subject that it was not worthy of intellectual effort. . . . Of course trauma is an untidy and heterogeneous subject, but its protean nature is precisely what makes it a challenge, and not to just one speciality or discipline either. There is something significant and exciting in this subject for every biomedical-related scientist, from the most basic micromolecular chemist to the most applied industrial engineer. There are highly relevant problems for behavioral scientists, biomechanical engineers, internists, pathologists, economists, hospital administrators, pharmacologists and computer scientists, to name a few of those who can add to the usual surgical and physiological approach. Everyone who can must be encouraged to contribute. We need a lot of help.[1]

The same could be said of work in medical, psychiatric, and other emergency care problems.

THE MAGNITUDE OF THE PROBLEM

U.S. national statistics underscore the magnitude of EMS needs. For example, accidents are the leading cause of death between the ages of one and thirty-seven and the fourth leading cause of death at all ages. Among accidental deaths, those due to motor vehicles constitute the leading cause for all age groups under seventy-five.[2] Trauma patients use more hospital days than all heart patients or obstetrical patients and more than four times as many hospital days as all cancer patients.[a] Studies suggest that mortality from vehicular accidents alone could be reduced by 15 to 20 percent by proper medical care at the scene of the accident or en route to an emergency facility—a saving nationally of approximately 11,000 lives.[3]

It is also estimated that from 5 to 20 percent of the 700,000 deaths resulting annually from heart disease—the leading cause of death at all ages—might be prevented if the public were educated to recognize the symptoms of heart attacks and if comprehensive EMS

[a]According to the National Academy of Sciences, "Each year more than 52 million U.S. citizens are injured, of whom more than 110,000 die, 11 million require bed care for a day or more, and 400,000 suffer lasting disability at a cost of nearly $3 billion in medical fees and hospital expenses and over $7 billion in lost wages. Those requiring hospitalization occupy an average of 65,000 beds for 22 million bed-days under the care of 88,000 hospital personnel. This hospital load is equivalent to 130 hospitals of 500 beds each." National Academy of Sciences, National Research Council, Division of Medical Sciences, Committee on Emergency Medical Services, "Roles and Resources of Federal Agencies in Support of Comprehensive Emergency Systems" (Washington, D.C.: National Research Council, March 1972), p. 3.

systems were in place throughout the nation.[4] Similarly, five thousand deaths each year from other causes such as poisonings, drownings, and drug overdoses might be prevented by immediate medical attention.[5] These are merely some of the major problems requiring effective emergency medical response which illustrate the potential payoff of a good EMS system.

DEFICIENCIES IN DELIVERY OF EMERGENCY CARE

In 1966 the National Academy of Sciences (NAS), after reviewing the care of trauma patients nationally, concluded that trauma was "the neglected disease of modern society."[6] After reexamining the national scene six years later, the NAS Committee on Emergency Medical Services concluded: "Emergency medical services is one of the weakest links in the delivery of health care in the nation."[7]

The Committee estimated that only 65 percent of the nation's ambulance attendants were trained to the advanced first aid level of the American National Red Cross and that 10 percent had no training in even the fundamentals of first aid. They noted that the majority of the nation's ambulances were of the hearse, limousine, or station wagon type (lacking adequate space to treat patients) and most did not have the basic medical equipment recommended by the American College of Surgeons. Many ambulances lacked radio communications even with their own dispatchers and few could establish direct contact with a physician, a hospital emergency department, or with police or fire personnel. In most parts of the country the citizen had no easily identifiable number to call to request emergency medical assistance, causing confusion and unnecessary delay in ambulance response.[8]

For the patient who reaches the hospital, emergency care has been complicated because so many Americans now utilize the emergency department (ED) for their nonurgent primary care. Studies show that the majority of ED patients do not require true emergency care and could be readily treated in nonacute primary care facilities. Only 5 percent or less of ED patients are critically ill or injured.[9] Few hospitals have successfully dealt with this problem and few areas have organized their capabilities to ensure that patients with special emergency problems, such as burns or spinal cord injuries, are taken to the best equipped facility.

Thus, in the early 1970s, although there were a few excellent EMS systems, most were fragmented, unorganized, and inadequate. This is explained in part because most physicians and health leaders as well as the public had not made EMS a priority. Many physicians who have been concerned with emergency care have focused on the hospital ED and not on the problems of prompt response to the emergency incident, quality care at the emergency scene, and on the need for upgraded ambulance services. For years, the hospital ED has been used as a spillover place to address problems which did not fit into the domain of physician specialists. In many teaching centers the result has been uneven delivery of care and inadequate teaching and supervision of interns and residents who rotate through the service.

THE EMERGING NATIONAL INTEREST IN EMS

During the past five years this gloomy picture has shown signs of change. A number of well-established organizations have intensified their efforts as professional and public interest in emergency care has increased. These organizations include: the American College of Surgeons, the American Heart Association, the National Safety Council, the American Academy of Orthopedic Surgeons, the American Medical Association, and the American Hospital Association. The Joint Commission on Accreditation of Hospitals has established new standards for emergency department accreditation. Many community colleges and junior colleges have become involved in the training of emergency medical technicians and other emergency medical personnel. Medical schools and nursing schools are placing greater emphasis on clinical emergency care problems, while emergency care organization, financing and evaluation issues are receiving increasing recognition as legitimate topics for health services research.

Several new organizations have been formed to address emergency care problems. These include: the American Trauma Society, the Emergency Department Nurses' Association, the American College of Emergency Physicians, the Society for Critical Care Medicine, the University Association for Emergency Medical Services, and the Society for Total Emergency Preparedness. Although each organization is concerned with different phases of emergency care, all have helped to raise the level of public awareness and concern about EMS—which is being translated into local action. Communities are establishing emergency medical councils and in some places are recognizing emergency medical care as a third public emergency service (with police and fire services) deserving of public support and standards of quality control.

THE INITIAL FEDERAL ROLE AND THE
U.S. DEPARTMENT OF TRANSPORTATION

Throughout much of the 1960s, the Division of Emergency Health Services of the Department of Health, Education and Welfare (HEW) was the only federal office that assumed significant responsibility for improving emergency medical services. This office operated with limited funding and authority and it focused its attention mostly on disaster preparedness and information dissemination.

The first significant evidence of congressional concern about emergency medical services was the enactment of the National Highway Safety Act of 1966. The Act authorized the U.S. Department of Transportation (DOT) to set guidelines for EMS. Under standard number 11 of the law, DOT has provided funds for: the purchase of ambulances and equipment, the installation of communications systems, the development and support of emergency medical technician training programs, and the development of statewide EMS plans.[10]

Under this law, federal funds have been allocated to each state on a block-grant basis and matched by state resources. Funds are distributed through each governor's highway safety representative for each of sixteen approved highway safety standards. In some states, EMS received few DOT dollars because other areas were given priority. In other states, EMS has been given high priority and has received considerable DOT funds.

One important result of DOT funding has been the emergence of a new health professional—the emergency medical technician-ambulance (EMT). With the contributions of several national organizations, including the National Academy of Sciences and the American Academy of Orthopedic Surgeons, an eighty-one-hour course was developed to teach emergency care fundamentals to ambulance personnel. A graduate of the course is designated an EMT I, according to the NAS, and this nomenclature has become well accepted.[11] The EMT is trained to maintain an airway, to treat hemorrhage and shock, to administer cardiopulmonary resuscitation, and to immobilize the patient with multiple injuries for transport to the hospital. In recent years, the EMT course has become accepted as the minimum training for a person who treats patients at the emergency scene or en route to a hospital via ambulance.

The growth of EMT training has been impressive. To date, the U.S. Department of Transportation estimates that 158,000 individuals have been trained as EMTs in all states. This constitutes 60 percent of the estimated 275,000 ambulance personnel that need training.[12] A twenty-hour refresher course has also been developed and is used widely. DOT standards recommend that EMTs take the refresher course at least every two years.

The Department of Transportation continues to support training programs as well as the purchase of vehicles and equipment, although its total EMS funds have decreased as HEW's role has increased (see pp. 11-14). DOT has supported the NAS in developing national standards for the EMT through a national registry that is giving a certification examination, and in developing training guidelines for the advanced EMT (EMT II). The EMT II is trained to perform cardiac defibrillation, read electrocardiograms at the emergency scene, administer certain drugs, and perform other advanced life-saving procedures, under the remote supervision of a physician.[13] DOT estimates that between 8,000 and 10,000 individuals have completed some type of EMT II (paramedic) training.[14] DOT also continues to support the Military Assistance in Safety and Traffic (MAST) program designed to use helicopters in EMS settings.[15]

REGIONAL MEDICAL PROGRAM ACTIVITY

Regional Medical Program (RMP) support for emergency medical services evolved in the early 1970s. Originally focused on heart disease, cancer, and stroke, the RMP legislation was expanded to include kidney and other related diseases. Under this authority, grants were made for a variety of purposes because decision-making about RMP funds was delegated to each of the fifty-six regional medical programs. Some excellent individual EMS efforts were undertaken using these funds, but there was no national RMP strategy in EMS and thus it is difficult to describe the national effort in this area. During the years 1970-72, $10.8 million were spent through RMP on some aspect of emergency medical services.[16] After considerable debate, the RMP legislation was not renewed in 1973.

FIVE HEW DEMONSTRATION PROJECTS

In 1968, an HEW advisory committee on traffic safety, under the chairmanship of Dr. Daniel P. Moynihan, concluded that the department should assume primary federal responsibility for emergency medical services.[17] In June 1970, Dr. Jesse Steinfeld, then Surgeon General of the U.S. Public Health Service, created a steering committee on emergency health care and injury control. That committee recommended that HEW consolidate all federal efforts in emergency medical services.[18]

Despite these activities, little progress was made until President Nixon's 1972 State of the Union Message which included a directive to HEW to "develop new ways of organizing emergency medical services and providing care to accident victims."[19] Two months later, the President stated: "I have already allocated $8 million in fiscal year 1972 to develop model systems and training programs and my budget proposes that $15 million be invested for additional demonstrations in fiscal year 1973."[20]

In response to this Presidential directive, the Health Services and Mental Health Administration (HSMHA) was designated as the lead agency within HEW and a program to develop five "total EMS systems" was launched. In June 1972, five contracts totaling $16 million were awarded to: the State of Arkansas, a three-county area of Southern California (San Diego), a seven-county area of Northeastern Florida (Jacksonville), the State of Illinois, and a seven-county area in Southeastern Ohio (Athens).[21]

As stated by an HEW official, the

> purpose of the EMS demonstration projects is not primarily to provide improved emergency services to the citizens of the respective areas, although this may be an important ancillary effect. The primary purpose is to develop and demonstrate various approaches to providing emergency medical care in a systematic and comprehensive manner so that other states and communities can look to these experiences in developing EMS systems for their citizens.[22]

A common thread running through much of the RMP programs and the HSMHA demonstration efforts was the emphasis on a regional approach to improving emergency medical care. It was increasingly accepted that all communities and hospitals could not provide comprehensive emergency medical services, and that our society simply could not afford competition between institutions and duplication of effort. The emphasis on shared resources and a regional approach to organizing EMS provided the basis upon which two recent national efforts in emergency care have been launched: The Robert Wood Johnson Foundation's program of Regional Emergency Medical Response Systems and the federal Emergency Medical Services Systems Act of 1973.

THE ROBERT WOOD JOHNSON FOUNDATION PROGRAM

Based on these experiences and cognizant of the growing national interest in EMS, The Robert Wood Johnson Foundation decided to make a major commitment to the field in the summer of 1972.[b] The Foundation's focus was on the front end of the emergency care system, namely the point of citizen access to emergency medical care. The Foundation recognized that in most parts of the country most citizens had no easily identifiable place to call when they needed emergency medical assistance. Further, in those few places where a well-publicized emergency medical telephone number existed, the person receiving the call seldom had training in how to deal with a request for emergency medical help. Even with trained dispatch personnel, the necessary assistance was often not readily mobilized because of the inability of the several emergency response agencies (ambulance, police, fire, and hospitals) to communicate effectively.

It was further evident that where communications systems did exist, many were constrained by political struggles and jurisdictional boundaries which prevented a patient from being taken to the most appropriate place for care. The Foundation concluded that emergency medical care could be strengthened through regionally based communications systems which integrated an area's emergency care resources into a comprehensive network of services.

Toward this end, $15 million was authorized for a nationwide program to encourage communities to develop regional emergency medical response systems based around visible access points.[c] The program received widespread attention in the press and 251 applications from forty-nine states and Puerto Rico were received.

Applications were reviewed by a multidisciplinary advisory committee of the NAS composed of prominent leaders in health and public affairs under the chairmanship of Dr. Robert Heyssel. After extensive site visits, the committee recommended forty-four regions for grant support of up to $400,000 each. Grants were announced in May 1974 and involve thirty-two states and Puerto Rico.

The grant program, which ends in 1977, is expected to yield considerable information concerning the problems of organizing regional systems of emergency care—information that should aid the implementation of the new national health planning legislation and other health planning.[23] Certain aspects of the program, particularly those related to regionalization, are being analyzed by the Rand Corpora-

[b]The Robert Wood Johnson Foundation emerged as a national philanthropy in 1972 as a result of a large bequest from the late Robert Wood Johnson. Located in Princeton, New Jersey, the Foundation has devoted its funds to improving access to primary health care in the United States.

[c]The program was announced on April 9, 1973, by Dr. David Rogers, president of the Foundation, and Dr. Philip Handler, president of the National Academy of Sciences, which is jointly administering the program. Guidelines from the Robert Wood Johnson Foundation program are contained in Appendix 1A.

tion. The NAS Committee and the Rand group expect to disseminate their findings by the end of 1977.

THE EMERGENCY MEDICAL SERVICES SYSTEMS ACT OF 1973

At the time of the development of the Robert Wood Johnson Foundation national initiative, congressional hearings were held on a proposed Emergency Medical Services Systems Act which took a similar regional and comprehensive systems approach to emergency care. The Act received support from many of the groups mentioned above, but after being approved by the House,[24] failed to pass the Senate.

A similar bill, entitled The Emergency Medical Services Systems Act of 1973, was adopted by both House and Senate after further public hearings in Washington, D.C., and California.[25] Amidst nearly unanimous public and professional support for the bill, the only opposition came from the administration.[26]

In August 1973, President Nixon vetoed the bill and stated:

At my direction, this administration has been engaged for the past two years in an effort to demonstrate the effectiveness of various types of emergency medical services which can be utilized by local communities. ... I strongly believe the federal role should be limited to such a demonstration effort, leaving states and communities free to establish the full range of emergency medical services systems that best suit their varying local needs.

By contrast, S-504 would establish a new federal grant program which would provide federal dollars to state and local governments for emergency medical services. The program would be a narrow categorical one thrusting the federal government into an area which is traditionally a concern of state and local governments and should remain under their jurisdiction.

The President added that federally defined objectives should not take precedence over locally determined priorities and the bill's authorization of $185 million was "far in excess" of what could be prudently spent, which would thus "mislead and disappoint the public."[27] Nixon also objected to the continued operation of inpatient facilities of the eight U.S. Public Health Service Hospitals, which was included as an amendment to the bill.

After narrowly failing to override the veto, new legislation was introduced (as Senate Bill 2410) with the Public Health Service

Hospital requirements deleted.[d] The Senate Committee on Labor and Public Welfare argued that the testimony before it revealed sufficient knowledge and experience to develop comprehensive EMS systems without further "demonstration" projects. The Committee again advocated a major federal EMS program and concluded that many communities would be unable to develop integrated regional EMS systems without federal technical assistance and funding.[28]

The Committee added that the provisions of S-2410 "do not impose an inflexible emergency medical services system upon the Nation's communities," but allow systems to be "suited to the particular medical emergency." The Committee further noted that there was no attempt in the legislation to "inflict any kind of rigid system on the communities" and that they were "well aware of the diversity of this Nation and of the individual characteristics of the Nation's communities."[29] It reiterated that "an effective emergency medical system must be designed to meet the individual characteristics of each community" and concluded that S-2410 provides this by calling upon each community to "come up with its own plan to provide the required components of a comprehensive system."[e]

With the provisions on the Public Health Service Hospitals deleted, Senate Bill 2410 was approved by the Senate and the House, and signed into law by the President as Public Law 93-154 in November 1973.[f] The purpose of the legislation has been to provide incentives to appropriate units of government to inventory their resources for providing comprehensive emergency medical services, identify the gaps in such services, seek to remedy these deficiencies through better coordination or utilization of existing resources, and develop the new components essential to the achievement of an integrated, comprehensive area EMS system.[g]

[d]The Senate voted to override by 77-16, but the House vote of 273-144 was 5 votes less than needed. Much of the House debate addressed the Public Health Service Hospitals issue.

[e]The Committee further stated that Senate 2410 was not a categorical approach, and that it required all communities to utilize any other sources of funds before these monies could be used. The Committee felt that the funding levels authorized were reasonable in light of the needs to improve emergency medical care in the country. Finally the Committee was critical of the support given the five HEW "demonstration" projects which had been awarded $8 million in fiscal 1972, but had been reduced in fiscal 1973 to $1.8 million. They concluded that the development of programs "must have a chance to become self-supporting," and that "communities should not be uncertain of the continued support necessary to build on the promising starts which have been made." Committee Report, p. 24.

[f]The legislation creates a new Title XII of the U.S. Public Health Service Act, and adds one new program of assistance to Title VII of that Act.

[g]According to the Committee Report, "The basic thrust of the Bill is to provide incentive payments for the development of a comprehensive and integrated

The Act, which authorized $185 million over three years, provides funds for "feasibility projects" (Section 1202), "establishment and initial operations of systems" (Section 1203), and "expansion and improvement" of systems (Section 1204).[h] The Act requires that state and local comprehensive health planning agencies have an opportunity to review and comment on all applications.

The legislation seeks to integrate the following fifteen elements into regional EMS systems: manpower, training, communications, transportation, facilities, critical care units, public safety agencies, consumer participation, accessibility to care, transfer of patients, standardized patient record-keeping, public information and education, independent review and evaluation, disaster linkages, and mutual aid agreements.[i]

The emphasis on regionalization is consistent with the Robert Wood Johnson Foundation national initiative. Indeed, eleven of the fifteen federal components appear in the Foundation guidelines. In defining the region, both programs emphasize existing natural patient care flow patterns rather than political or jurisdictional boundaries.[j] While the Robert Wood Johnson Foundation program has stressed the prehospital phase of the system using communications as a catalyst for change, HEW has emphasized improved inhospital capabilities, often using categorization of hospital emergency departments as a strategy for implementation.

In fiscal year 1974, HEW distributed $17 million to eighty-eight grantees under the EMS Systems Act. In fiscal year 1975, HEW

system with maximum reliance for funding placed on acquisition of funds and resources under other federal programs (especially for facilities, health manpower training, and transportation and equipment) through the division of Emergency Medical Programs, Department of Transportation, and MAST, and on the generation of local funds." Committee Report, p. 14.

[h]Regarding appropriated funds, a legislative formula required: 15 percent for 1202 in FY'74 and '75, 60 percent for 1203 in FY'74 and '75, 75 percent in FY'76, and 25 percent for 1204 in each fiscal year.

[i]A more detailed description of the HEW program is included in Appendix 1B.

[j]HEW program guidelines implementing the Act define a regional EMS system as "one that is geographically described by the existing natural patient care flow patterns. It must be large enough in size and population to provide definitive care services to the majority of general, emergent and critical patients. Where care deficiencies of a highly sophisticated nature exist within the region, arrangements must be made for obtaining these patient care services in an adjoining region. Various counties and cities will need to be grouped and the region may have to be larger than the boundaries of an Areawide Comprehensive Health Planning Agency. It is the definition of the EMS regional delivery area with its patient distribution patterns that is the essential issue." U.S. Department of Health, Education and Welfare, Emergency Medical Services Systems Program Guidelines (Revised February 1975), p. 14. (Hereafter cited as HEW Guidelines.)

awarded an additional $32.2 million to 114 regions in forty-seven states, and the District of Columbia.[k] The Department subsequently announced grants totaling $29.1 million for fiscal year 1976 to fifty-two recipients in thirty-four states, the District of Columbia, and Puerto Rico.

According to Dr. David Boyd, director of the Division of Emergency Medical Services in HEW, the agency has divided the country into over 300 EMS regions. Thus, over a third of the nation has now received federal support under the Act for developing basic life support (BLS) regional emergency medical services systems.[l]

THE INCREASING STATE ROLE IN EMS

Concurrent with the major foundation and federal efforts in emergency care has been a growth of interest and commitment at the state level. Nowhere is this more apparent than the widespread enactment of state legislation relating to emergency medical services during the past four years.

According to the National Emergency Medical Services Information Clearinghouse (NEMSIC) at the University of Pennsylvania, twenty-one states have adopted "comprehensive" emergency medical services legislation in the past four years. Typically, these laws include the creation or expansion of a state division of emergency

[k]Of the $32 million awarded in fiscal '75, fifty-six grants ($4.6 million) were Section 1202 planning grants, forty-seven ($19.5 million) were Section 1203 implementation grants, and eleven ($8.1 million) were Section 1204 expansion or improvement grants.

[l]Section 1205 of the Act provides funds for EMS research. Under the direction of Dr. Lawrence Rose in the Health Resources Administration, grants and contracts totaling $3 million in fiscal '74, and $4.5 million in fiscal '75 were awarded. According to Dr. Rose, the quality of EMS research has improved, and is now competitive with other health services research projects. As comprehensive regional emergency medical systems are developed, important questions about implementation will appear and will require research.

Under Title VII of the Health Professions Education Systems Act, thirty-nine grants totaling $4.5 million were awarded for training in emergency medical services in fiscal 1975. The funds were limited to EMT training at both the basic and advanced levels. A contract was awarded to the National Registry for Emergency Medical Technicians to develop materials to examine and test emergency medical technicians in various clinical procedures.

As required under the law, an Interagency Committee on Emergency Medical Services has been formed to coordinate the many federal programs related to EMS. The Committee has five public members and representatives from twenty-two federal agencies. The law also required a detailed study of potential legal barriers to improve EMS, including such issues as: malpractice, good samaritan laws, and licensure statutes.

medical services (usually under its Department of Health) with licensing and standard-setting authority, and authorization for state or regional EMS councils to develop EMS plans and provide continuing advice. Many also include development of a state EMS communications plan, authorization for incorporated cities or counties to contract for or operate ambulance services and authority to categorize hospital emergency departments.[30]

Other states have limited their legislation to ambulance services. These statutes usually include minimum standards relating to training of ambulance personnel, types of equipment and vehicles, and some requirements regarding licensure of ambulance providers. Other laws provide exemption for physicians, nurses, and EMTs from malpractice liability, and modify licensure provisions to permit advanced EMTs to function up to their level of training at the emergency scene by acting under physician supervision and control.[m]

In addition to increased legislative activity, several states have begun to appropriate more funds for EMS. For example, Connecticut, which had previously allocated few funds for EMS, authorized $275,000 in 1973.

EMS COMMUNICATIONS AND
FCC DOCKET #19880

The importance of communications as the link to bring together all various components of an EMS system has been recognized, but until recently, the nation's communications capability fell far short of the needs. In 1967 the President's Commission on Law Enforcement and Administration of Justice recommended that a single number be established for reporting police emergencies and in 1968, the American Telephone and Telegraph Company announced that it would reserve the digits 911 for emergency use nationally. As interest in 911 developed, it became clear that the number could be used for fire and medical emergencies as well. In March 1973, the Office of Telecommunications Policy in the executive office of the President issued a national policy statement which recognized the benefits of 911 and encouraged its nationwide adoption.[31]

In the past, emergency medical services have suffered because the number of radio frequencies authorized by the Federal Communica-

---

[m]Other states have passed laws to implement standard 11 of the Highway Safety Act of 1966. Understandably, this legislation tends to focus less on comprehensive EMS systems and more on driver education, alcohol abuse education and prevention, elimination of road hazards, and other highway related programs.

tions Commission for EMS has been limited. (The Federal Communications Commission has regulatory authority to allocate civilian radio frequencies.) Traditionally, priority for emergency radio use has been concentrated on law enforcement and firefighting activities.

In November 1973, the Office of Telecommunications Policy submitted a detailed study of emergency medical communications to the FCC. The report describes the communications problems facing EMS and notes that the Federal Communications Commission provided frequencies in the 30-50 mhz and in the 155.13-155.430 mhz bands for base and mobile operations for general emergency medical radio communications. The report concludes that these frequencies (thirty-two in number) are allocated as a part of the special emergency radio service which means that EMS must share with disaster relief agencies, school buses, beach patrols, and common carrier standby and repair facilities.[n]

The report points out that there are other limitations to EMS use including the "doughnut rule," which prohibits the same frequency use by a station located within forty miles of another station.[32] According to this study, there were 11,721 licensees for the thirty-two frequencies available for EMS communications or a national average of 366 licensees per frequency.

The Office of Telecommunications Policy report contained many recommendations for changing the FCC rules. The most fundamental recommendation was that the FCC establish a medical services category in the "special emergency radio service," to eliminate the competition and crowding outlined above.

The OTP report and comments on it received from over 200 sources led to the adoption of Docket #19880 by the Federal Communications Commission in July 1974.[33] The new FCC rules provide for a medical services category, expand the licensure eligibility provisions, make available several additional UHF frequencies (for both dispatch and telemetry), and augment VHF capability. The rules support the development of coordinated, "areawide" EMS communications systems and the establishment of central dispatch and control centers.

The HEW program guidelines issued in support of the Emergency Medical Services Systems Act support the position taken in Docket #19880. The HEW regulations state:

[n]Office of Telecommunications Policy, "Communications in Support of Emergency Medical Services," Washington, D.C., November 1973. The study, which was carried out by the Interdepartment Radio Advisory Committee (IRAC), became known as the IRAC Report. (Hereafter cited as IRAC Report.)

the system should include a system command and control center which would be responsible for establishing those communication channels and allocating those public resources essential to the most effective and efficient EMS management of the immediate problem. . . . The essentials of such a command and control center are that (a) all requests for system response are directed to the center; (b) all system resource response is directed from the center; and (c) all system liaison with other public safety and emergency response systems is coordinated from the center.[34]

Thus FCC Docket #19880 has not only made available the needed additional UHF and VHF frequencies, but it enhances the development of regional emergency medical response systems as advocated in the Robert Wood Johnson Foundation and HEW programs.

PHYSICIAN SPECIALIZATION IN EMERGENCY MEDICINE

Physician interest in emergency medical care has grown considerably, as evidenced by the increasing leadership of many physicians in organizing EMS systems, and by others in the full-time practice of emergency medicine. Such interest is reflected by the growth of the American College of Emergency Physicians established in 1968 and by the recent development of residency training programs in emergency medicine.

The first emergency medicine residency program was established at the University of Cincinnati in 1970. The American College of Emergency Physicians now lists thirty-two residency programs in emergency medicine, most of which are located in community hospitals and are two years in length. The residencies have grown in response to the increased use of full time physicians in the emergency departments of community hospitals. Many hospitals are now looking for a physician "specialist" in emergency medicine.

In 1975, the American Medical Association's House of Delegates recommended to their Council on Medical Education (CME) that emergency medicine emerge as a new specialty with accreditation and certification mechanisms comparable to other specialty areas. In 1976, the American College of Emergency Physicians and the University Association of Emergency Medical Services jointly filed a formal reqest to the AMA's CME and the American Board of Medical Specialties (ABMS) for such recognition, and this is being considered by the Liaison Committee on Specialty Boards (a joint committee of the AMA's CME and the ABMS).[35]

In 1975, two academic medical centers established special programs designed to develop faculty to teach clinical and nonclinical aspects of emergency medicine. These programs provide exposure to management, financing, organization, and evaluation issues. (The programs are located at the Johns Hopkins University School of Medicine and the University of California School of Medicine, San Francisco.)

THE STATE OF EMS RESEARCH

The increase in EMS activity nationally has raised many issues that need further research. A comprehensive review of EMS research was conducted in 1974 by the Bureau of Public Administration at the University of Tennessee. The project, under the direction of Dr. Hyram Plaas, was supported by the National Science Foundation as one of a series of nineteen projects on the evaluation of policy-related research in the field of municipal systems, operation, and services.[36]

The project attempted to identify information gaps in EMS research and to inform EMS decisionmakers of existing valid research that might be useful in making policy choices. The study identified 1,620 EMS-related items of which 592 were research or research-related studies.

Some of the major findings of this review were:

(1) There is no area of emergency medical services which has a sufficient research base. . . . (2) There are very few research centers with a continuing interest and capability for the conduct of basic or policy related research in emergency medical services. . . . (3) Past and present funding sources and processes discourage the development of quality proposals for basic and policy related research particularly that conducted within the settings of higher educational institutions. . . . (5) Demonstration projects have not proven fruitful to date as research mechanisms due to design problems, the absence of comparability, the absence of the establishment of control groups, the emphasis upon program implementation, a lack of tested and validated performance measures, and a compulsion to demonstrate success. (6) A major investment is needed in the development of research methodology and design in EMS. First priority in this effort should be given to the development and refinement of performance measures and to the testing of patient outcomes. (7) A high-priority in EMS policy related research should be placed upon studies concerned with organizational management of EMS systems. These studies should emphasize policy decision making, program management, and clinical process levels, and should aid in the development of alternative organization and management tools. Significant progress has been made in research related to emergency medical transportation, but the research in hospital emergency departments is too heavily focused on descriptive studies of patient characteristics and patient utilization.[37]

In summary, the Tennessee review stresses the importance of continuing research during a time when increased implementation dollars are available for EMS.

WASHINGTON UPDATE—1976

The importance of EMS as a national health issue received a visible boost at a White House Conference held on January 6, 1976, during which many recent developments in the field were reviewed. At the conference, President Ford described the recent HEW EMS initiative as "an excellent program" and concluded that the "federal demonstration projects had proven their worthiness" in saving lives. He called it "a program that is totally justified" and stated that "it illustrates that people at the local level are best able to decide how federal monies should be spent." However, the President indicated his opposition to continuing categorical federal programs and his preference for bloc grants to states.[38] This strategy, termed the Financial Assistance for Health Care Act, was announced by the President a few weeks later in his State of the Union Address.

Later in January 1976, hearings were held before the Senate's Subcommittee on Health of the Committee on Labor and Public Welfare to consider extending the Emergency Medical Services Systems Act of 1973 which was scheduled to expire in 1976. Testifying for the administration, Dr. Theodore Cooper, Assistant Secretary for Health, stated that the EMS Act had "successfully demonstrated emergency medical services techniques to local communities" and had "resulted in substantial numbers of lives saved." After concluding that "a great deal has been accomplished to improve the awareness and the delivery" of EMS systems, Dr. Cooper asserted that continuation of the existing legislation was "no longer necessary."[39] Instead he urged the adoption of the President's bloc grant approach while assuring that existing federal EMS grantees be guaranteed phase out support over three years.

In contrast, all public testimony and statements from Committee members strongly favored continuing the EMS legislation. For example, Senator Alan Cranston warned that the "systematic regional approach" which was "the basic justification" for the legislation would probably be lost under the bloc grant strategy.[40]

In the fall of 1975, the U.S. General Accounting Office conducted a preliminary assessment of EMS activity under the 1973 Act based on a review of twelve HEW grantees. In support of the program, the GAO concluded that sufficient data were available to show that communities had been able to upgrade their EMS resources and that it was "fair to assume" this had "resulted in some decrease in mortality and morbidity." However, the GAO noted that truly integrated regional EMS systems were being established with difficulty because regional management entities often lacked control over their system's resources. This was causing delays in obtaining local commitments to provide operating funds after the grant period, and in obtaining agreements concerning the optimal number and location of ambulances, categorization of emergency facilities, operation of regional communications systems (with central command and control authority), and the use of standardized patient record keeping forms. The GAO concluded that changes in the proposed legislation might overcome these barriers and urged HEW to better coordinate its efforts with other federal agencies who were also involved in EMS.[41]

Subsequently, on February 12, 1976, the Office of Management and Budget re-affirmed the HEW position opposing enactment of the extension legislation. Instead they urged the adoption of President Ford's Financial Assistant for Health Care Act which they believed would give states "the flexibility necessary to support . . . projects tailored to the particular needs of the State and its subdivisions."[42]

However, as expected, the Congress voted favorably on the extension bill titled the "Emergency Medical Services Amendments of 1976." Although the new Act makes numerous changes in the 1973 Act (including several recommended by the GAO), the basic approach of developing regional EMS systems containing 15 components remains intact.[43] During 1977 through 1979, the bill authorized $200 million for systems development, $15 million for research, $40 million for training, and $14 million for a new burn injury program. Undoubtedly with some ambivalence, President Ford signed the bill into law on October 21, 1976.

A DECADE OF CHANGE

During the past decade, EMS has emerged from a minor and obscure position to one of high visibility and activity. The recognition at national, state, and local levels of the importance of improved emergency medical services and the role of emergency ambulance care as an important public service is both striking and encouraging.

It is too early to assess whether the many regional systems now under development will have the impact promised by their advocates or will become financially self-sufficient once Federal funding ends. Answers to the first question will depend upon the ability of researchers and analysts to measure and assess the actual impact of such systems. Answers to the second will depend on whether local governments are persuaded that quality emergency medical care is a priority public service that is worthy of continued financial support. It may be close to another decade before we know the true pay-offs of the efforts of the past ten years.

Appendix 1A

Excerpts from the Robert Wood Johnson Foundation's National Grants Program of Regional Emergency Medical Response Systems (April 9, 1973)

IV. MINIMUM REQUIREMENTS FOR ELIGIBILITY

To be eligible, the program applicant must give evidence of capacity and intention of meeting the following minimum requirements within a one-year period of receiving a grant:

A. *Central and immediate citizen access to the emergency medical system.* It is essential that the general public have access to all forms of emergency medical care through a single telephone number. Calling this number would put any person in contact with a central emergency medical dispatch agency. This should be accessible from all telephones, including pay phones where it is preferable that a coin *not* be required to reach the emergency number.

B. *Central control of communications with a single regional institution assigned responsibility for dispatch and coordination of emergency medical vehicles and services and for collection of data necessary for effective internal management and monitoring of the system.* The proposal must specify the agency that would have overall *authority and responsibility* for the operation of the emergency medical dispatch system. The proposal must provide clear evidence of cooperation and agreement to participate from all appropriate agencies.

C. *Prompt central medical dispatching of appropriate emergency care to the scene of the emergency and direction of patients to appropriate medical facilities.* This involves a trained central medical emergency dispatcher (CMED) who responds to notification of emergency situations via telephone or radio from private citizens, public agencies, or governmental institutions. It is expected that the CMED would:

1. Establish priorities and initiate appropriate response of the emergency medical system. If emergency medical assistance is needed, this response would include:

   a. dispatch of an ambulance with trained personnel and appropriate equipment,

   b. communication with those personnel en route to the scene,

   c. communication with related agencies when necessary,

   d. communication with the ambulance personnel after arrival at the scene to obtain such information as: the types and number of victims, the need for additional vehicles or equipment, and the need for ancillary and backup medical facilities.

2. Where appropriate and feasible, facilitate patient-related clinical communication between personnel at (or en route to and from) the scene and physicians or other medical professionals.

3. Based on information received from the scene and from the relevant medical facilities, direct the transport of the patient or patients to appropriate facilities.

The CMED agency would assume two additional vital functions:

4. Continuous and current assessment of the areawide emergency vehicle status and other relevant medical facilities.

5. Initial and backup response to other agencies involved in disaster situations.

The CMED agency would necessarily require functional integration with the daily activities of police departments, fire departments, civil defense, rescue units, utility companies, and other involved agencies. It would include the cooperative arrangements needed for integrating these emergency services into an effective emergency preparedness and response system. It would also identify the functional requirements for communications among the relevant agencies in the emergency system and establish procedures for routine interagency information exchange.

D. *Adequately trained dispatch, ambulance and other health personnel.*

1. All central medical emergency dispatchers must complete the Department of Transportation Emergency Medical Dispatcher course or its equivalent before assuming this role (see enclosed booklet). As soon as feasible, all CMEDs should complete the 81-hour Department of Transportation Emergency Medical Technician/Ambulance course or its equivalent.
2. The great majority of ambulance personnel shall have completed the 81-hour DOT EMT/Ambulance course or its equivalent by the end of the two-year funding period.
3. As soon as feasible, advanced emergency medical training should be made available to emergency medical technicians, nurses, and physicians.

E. *Prompt and appropriate emergency system capacity.* This would include:
1. Twenty-four hour availability of properly designed and equipped vehicles staffed by trained emergency medical technicians.
2. Adequately staffed and equipped 24-hour hospital or clinic emergency department capability, with substantive progress toward regionalization and categorization.
3. Adequate communications equipment for transmission of voice information between hospitals, ambulances and the CMED agency.
4. Hospital specialized care capabilities (e.g., burn units, coronary care units, trauma unit, poison control centers).

F. *Access to adequate radio channels and telephone lines for a comprehensive emergency medical services system.*
G. *Assurance that after the two years of support, the program would become self-sufficient, with its subsequent operational expenditures becoming part of the budgets of the applicant or other agencies.*

V. PRIORITIES

Among proposals meeting all of the minimum requirements for eligibility stated above, priority will be given to those including the following characteristics (not ranked in the order presented):

A. Those which offer greatest potential impact in reducing mortality and disability.
B. Those which provide for the most effective use of other public and private resources (including maximal use of existing com-

munications equipment, existing community planning mechanisms, and existing training programs) which, as a result, are able to apply for reduced funding levels below the maximum of $400,000.

C. Those which demonstrate strong linkages and coordination with other emergency services and planning agencies, such as police and fire departments, hospitals, comprehensive health planning agencies, regional emergency services planning councils, and civil defense agencies.

D. Those which demonstrate consistency with state, local or regional emergency medical services plans if they exist.

E. Those which would serve regions which encompass a large geographic (e.g., multi-county) area or large population (e.g., metropolitan) size.

F. Those which would serve regions that can provide evidence of hospital commitment to develop and implement a plan of categorization of hospital emergency capabilities by the end of the two-year funding period.

G. Those which would serve regions which can demonstrate the commitment to provide, within the two-year funding period, identification plaques on telephones to aid the caller to reach the CMED when emergency assistance is needed and to provide coin-free pay telephones for dialing the central medical emergency dispatch number (such as 911).

H. Those which provide training in emergency medical services for physicians, nurses, and other involved health personnel.

I. Those which provide a plan to inform and educate the public in the region of the proper use of the emergency medical system and citizen responsibility in emergency care.

J. Those which make appropriate provision for three levels of function: routine transport of non-emergency patients, care and transport of patients needing basic emergency medical assistance, and care and transport of patients requiring advanced medical assistance.

K. Those giving evidence that, when new ambulances or equipment are purchased, they are in accord with National Academy of Sciences guidelines and Department of Transportation standards.

L. Those which demonstrate the development and operation of such a system with the greatest cost effectiveness.

✳ *Appendix 1B*

Excerpts from the Emergency Medical Services Systems Act of 1973— Program Guidelines*

CHAPTER III—SPECIAL PROGRAM GUIDANCE

This Chapter summarizes the essential emergency medical care issues, the regionalization of EMS and the 15 mandatory program requirements for EMS system planning, operation and management. Applicants should give careful consideration to these topics in the written application. It also describes some of the factors that DHEW will consider in assessing exceptional financial need.

A. Emergency Medical Care Issues

The central theme of the EMSS Act was to develop systems of emergency medical care that would significantly decrease current death and disability rates. The intent of the EMSS Act is to initiate regional planning and integrate the 15 mandatory components so as to provide the essential EMS services for all emergency patients.

The current EMS patient problem is compounded by the 50 million citizens who access the system each year. At least eighty (80) percent of these patients cannot be considered "true emergencies." Fifteen (15) percent are real emergencies which require urgent care (i.e., minor trauma, infectious disease and other acute general medical and surgical problems). The remaining five (5) percent are the critically ill and injured patients. This last group was not salvageable

---

*Prepared by the Division of Emergency Medical Services, Health Services Administration, West Hyattsville, Maryland, 1974.

a few years ago, but these lives can be saved today if initial definitive and rehabilitative care is given in time and the patient is moved through the system to obtain essential services.

The clinical critical capabilities that have been identified in several Federal EMS system demonstrations and other regional EMS projects are (1) care of accident victims, (2) specific care of the burn victim, (3) acute coronary care for the myocardial infarction, (4) care of high risk infants, (5) patient management for poisonings, drug overdose, acute alcohol intoxication and (6) psychiatric emergencies. There are many other emergent conditions (stroke, diseases, unique medical and surgical emergencies) which the EMS system will encounter. However, they do not lend themselves, as well, for regional planning and operation of models.

Specific planning for regional EMS response to these particular critical care groups will mean that all critical medical emergencies will receive better care, and will benefit from, sound regional EMS systems planning and operation. Other emergent conditions, because of their relative lower incidence, and community appreciation, do not lend themselves to initiating regional EMS planning and operation.

Certain local occupational hazards might also be addressed with a goal toward prevention. These special patient groups provide each regional system an opportunity to develop evaluation criteria for systems performance on patient outcome.

Each regional plan should include a description for the general routine emergent and non-emergent patient care delivery. It should include a detailed explanation of care patterns for critical groups by identifying the patient treatment needs as well as all of the systems operational elements. These care patterns will depend upon the clinical patient demands, the sophistication of transportation capability, level of care during transportation, delivery to a categorized general hospital or designated critical care facility and migration into the rehabilitation phase. These patient care patterns must be established with backup relationships. There is need for written arrangements among the various provider elements which emphasize sound area-wide care for an EMS system.

A general discussion of the emergency problems, including overloading of emergency facilities, is appropriate for the non-emergent patients, but is not helpful as the sole description of the EMS operation. General EMS problems exist in most communities and a large number of patients visit emergency facilities for general health care (non-emergent problems). However, it is the critically ill and injured that must be addressed in terms of life saving EMS systems design implementation and operations.

When one becomes seriously ill or injured he does it in a rather specific way. Patients become injured. They have heart attacks. They are burned. They have problems with birth. They are poisoned with alcohol, drugs, or other toxiants. They have emotional disturbances of varying degrees of psychiatric instability. Therefore, the planning of EMS systems must consider the general population and all identifiable and significant patient groups and problems that occur within the geographic regional area.

An indepth knowledge of the demography, epidemiology and clinical requirements associated with the critical patient groups is mandatory. This relationship must be spelled out in the application in order to address and integrate the 15 components in the regional EMS planning.

In many circumstances the initial patient access, response and transportation considerations are general in nature until the severity of the patient (diagnostic-specific) problem becomes clarified. As soon as this clarification develops, a rather specific patient treatment plan can be developed to include the pre-hospital, in-hospital, inter-hospital periods and as appropriate the specialty care unit and the specific rehabilitation services for a specific illness or injury.

It is a fairly well accepted position across the country that initial medical care for all of these well identifiable patient (non-emergent, emergent, and critical) groups can be improved and patients can be salvaged by EMS systems. The redesign of existing EMS capabilities will include organization and operational changes. There must be adaptations of treatments in the pre-hospital and inter-hospital phases with proper modification of technical and specific equipment that will enable paraprofessionals and professionals to manage and treat clinical problems in urban, rural and wilderness areas.

After there is an established BLS system in the region, progression to an ALS system is anticipated. This logical expansion of EMS must be based on the capability of the EMS region to assemble the critical elements of advanced medical equipment and to train people to provide complex and sophisticated care.

It is these health care aspects that must be stressed in EMS planning and operations. Applicants should prepare the application with fairly detailed narratives of what the emergency care situation is now and how they plan to change that situation during the grant period. For example, describe how the proposed EMS system would respond for an accident victim in a certain locale. How the patient would be evaluated and transported to an appropriate hospital or critical care unit. Describe how high risk infants born in a hospital would be evaluated by a physician/nurse, transported from the hospital to a designated neonatal high risk center within that region or in an adjoining region.

This preplanning of care arrangements and specified facilities, for these critical patients is essential to an EMS System.

B. Regionalization of Emergency
Medical Services

A regional EMS system is one that is geographically described by the existing natural patient care flow patterns. It must be large enough in size and population to provide definitive care services to the majority of general, emergent and critical patients. Where care deficiencies of a highly sophisticated nature exist within the region, arrangements must be made for obtaining these patient care services in an adjoining region. Various counties and cities will need to be grouped and the region may have to be larger than the boundaries of an Areawide Comprehensive Health Planning Agency. It is the definition of the EMS regional delivery area with its patient distribution patterns that is the essential issue.

The regional operational organization must attempt to pull together the EMS services within these medical-geographic arrangements. The planning and evaluation process must be based upon sound clinical considerations and with State and inter-regional relationships being maintained. In these EMS regions the provider elements within the geographic area will need to work together to solve mutual problems. The EMS Council must be developed with advisory input into these regional EMS programs and their relationship to other regional or State health authorities.

The EMS region must be contiguous with the adjoining regions. Regional planners should recognize that population in the fringe areas of a region may need to develop dual plans and allow for inter-communications with adjoining regional EMS plans and operations. A coordination mechanism should be developed between intra-state regions and inter-state regions.

The EMS system must be integrated through an appropriate regional organization so that the total resources can be effectively utilized to meet the needs of the geographical area. The financial resources of the area must be sufficient and mobilized to develop and sustain the EMS system operation. The EMS system must be interfaced with the total health care delivery system for the region. The EMS system resources must be linked to local disaster organizations in order to respond to sporadic high intensity needs such as a natural disaster within the regional service area and joining service areas.

The role for the health professionals, hospital associations, and EMS councils is to consider the critical professional services required to establish community wide and regional care programs, to recruit the EMS professionals, to affirm the economic base, and to provide community access to these emergency care resources when needed.

C. EMS System Components

The EMSS Act of 1973 requires that plans developed and systems established, expanded, and improved with funds under this Act address the following components:

1. Manpower
2. Training
3. Communications
4. Transportation
5. Facilities
6. Critical Care Units
7. Public Safety Agencies
8. Consumer Participation
9. Accessibility to Care
10. Transfer of Patients
11. Standard Medical Record-Keeping
12. Public Information and Education
13. Evaluation
14. Disaster Linkage
15. Mutual Aid Agreements

In reviewing applications for funding the DHEW shall consider these 15 components as mandatory. If an applicant determines that one or more of these components are not appropriate or non-achievable within an areawide system, then justification must be provided to show an alternative system configuration which meets the intent of the Act. The intent is to address each component as is appropriate for the special geography and medical conditions of the region.

Guidance on the Scope and Specificity of Each Component Is Set Forth Below for Applicant Assistance.

1. *Manpower*—An adequate number of health professionals, allied health professionals and other health personnel, including ambulance personnel, with appropriate training and experience.

This means sufficient numbers of all types of personnel to provide EMS on a 24-hour a day basis, 7 days a week, within the service area of the system. These manpower needs must be addressed even if funds are not requested for their support or training.

The EMS system must emphasize recruitment of veterans of the Armed Forces with military training and experience in health care fields and of appropriate public safety personnel in such areas. The major manpower elements to be considered are as follows:

- First Responders—fire, police, and other public safety elements
- Communicators—EMS/Resources Dispatcher
- Emergency Medical Technician—Ambulance (EMT-A)
- Emergency Medical Technician—Paramedic (EMT-Paramedic)
- Registered Nurses—Emergency Department
- Registered Nurses—Critical Care Units
- Physician—Emergency
- Physician—Specialty (medical, surgical, pediatric, psychiatry)
- EMS Systems Director—Physician, Administrator
- EMS System Coordinators

2. *Training*—The provision for appropriate training (including clinical training) and continuing education programs which (1) are coordinated with other programs in the system's service area which provide similar training and education and (2) emphasize recruitment and necessary training of veterans of the Armed Forces with military training and experience in health care fields and of appropriate public safety personnel in such areas.

"Appropriate public safety personnel" includes police, firemen, lifeguards, park rangers and other public employees charged with maintaining the public safety.

3. *Communications*—Provisions for linking the personnel, facilities, and equipment of the system by a central communications system so that requests for emergency health care services will be handled by a communications facility which (1) utilizes emergency telephonic screening, (2) utilizes or will utilize the universal emergency telephone number 911, and (3) will have direct communication connections and interconnections with the personnel, facilities, and equipment of the system and with other appropriate emergency medical services systems.

The system should include a system command and control center which would be responsible for establishing those communication channels and allocating those public resources essential to the most effective and efficient EMS management of the immediate problem. The center should have the necessary equipment and facilities to permit immediate interchange of information essential for the system's resource management and control. The essentials of such a command and control center are that (a) all requests for system response are directed to the center; (b) all system resource response is directed from the center; and (c) all system liaison with other public safety and emergency response systems is coordinated from the center.

The EMS communications system must address access, allocation of resources, management (central dispatch) and medical control for basic life support and advanced life support.

The communication elements should include:

Access providing public interface system to emergency resource system
- 911
- Alternative single access number

Resource Management Function
- Central Dispatch
- Coordination of EMS and other public services

Medical Control
- Medical communications to hospital for triage, diagnosis and treatment

Hospital to Mobile
- Basic voice
- Basic voice/Advanced biomedical telemetry

Hospital to Hospital
- Basic voice
- Advanced biomedical telemetry (optional)

Operational experience with "911" systems providing access to police, fire, and EMS has shown that approximately 85% of the incoming calls involve police services; 10% fire services, and 5% emergency medical services. Applicants should thoroughly investigate the implementation and use of 911 as the community central access number. Funds under this Act may be used to assist implementation of a 911 system commensurate with the level of EMS usage.

Applicants should, during the planning phase, develop a 911 implementation plan. If the community is not prepared for immediate 911 implementation, the communications plan should set forth a time at which 911 will be reexamined.

DHEW also supports the ultimate transfer of EMS system communications to the UHF band. Neither EMS system communications planning nor equipment procurement in other than the UHF band will be encouraged. Generally, it is the policy of DHEW to support new EMS communications systems which are designed to operate in the UHF band. Grant applications and EMS system planning documents will be carefully evaluated in accordance with this policy. However, where the requested project involves completion of a partially completed system, and after a case by case evaluation of the proposed methods of interface between UHF and VHF systems, DHEW may support communications in the VHF band.

4. *Transportation*—This component shall include an adequate number of necessary ground, air and water vehicles and other transportation facilities properly equipped to meet the transportation and EMS characteristics of the system area. Such vehicles and facilities must meet appropriate standards relating to location, design, performance, and equipment; and the operators and other personnel for such vehicles and facilities must meet appropriate training and experience requirements.

The elements of transportation should include:

Ground—Basic Life Support Elements
- Ambulance vehicles meeting DOT/GSA specifications and including equipment recommended by the American College of Surgeons, DHEW and DOT.
- Radio communication providing 2 way voice/for vehicle control and for medical control and consultation
- At least two EMT-As
- Locations permitting (for 95% of all calls) a maximum of a 30 minute response time in rural areas
- Locations permitting (for 95% of all calls) a maximum of a 10 minute response time in metropolitan areas

Ground—Advanced Life Support Elements
- All elements of a ground Basic Life Support component, plus personnel trained beyond the EMT-A level to address specific clinical items in medical service plan
- Extra communications to provide advanced biomedical telemetry
- Extra equipment

Air
- Helicopters
  —Primary response—unique use depending on geographical constraints
  —Secondary response—30–150 mile transport radius

- Fixed Wing
  —Greater response for 150 mile transport radius
- Water
  —Special geographical considerations
- Snow Mobile
  —Special geographical considerations

5. *Facilities*—This component shall include an adequate number of easily accessible emergency medical service facilities which are collectively capable of providing service on a continuous (24 hour a day, 7 days a week) basis, which have appropriate standards relating to capacity, location, personnel, and equipment, and which are coordinated with other health care facilities of the system.

Elements for facilities consideration include:

- Regional categorization with accepted State or national criteria with at least one Category II hospital providing 24-hour physician coverage in the emergency department in each EMS region.
- Regional EMS Advisory Groups to plan and carry out the categorization plan. These groups should include hospital administrators, physicians, nurses, other providers and health system planners.
- Regional plans for mutual agreement of categories, use of critical care units, systems linkages and resource sharing.

6. *Critical Care Units*—This component requires providing access (including appropriate transportation) to specialized critical medical care units. These units should be in the number and variety necessary to meet the demands of the service area. If there are no such units in the EMS region, then the system will provide access to units in neighboring areas if feasible in terms of time and distance.

Specialized critical medical care units should include trauma intensive care units, burn centers, spinal cord centers, and detoxification centers, coronary care units, high risk infant units, drug overdose and psychiatric centers and others as appropriate.

Appropriate transportation means a vehicle equipped and staffed with at least two EMTs or more highly trained personnel to administer to the patient's in-transit needs.

A twofold issue here is the availability of critical care service units within the EMS region or in neighboring regions. Specialty care services should address an adequate number of beds in the region or access to critical care units in neighboring areas. An operational plan for utilization of critical care units should be developed, including trained personnel, equipment and transportation.

The EMS system should include the development of professional advisory groups to work with EMS programs to insure that these critical services be utilized and interrelate across political boundaries.

7. *Public Safety Agencies*—Provisions must be made for effective utilization of appropriate personnel, facilities, and equipment of each public safety agency in the area.

"Effective utilization" means the integration of public safety agencies into standard EMS and disaster operating procedures of the areawide system. It also includes the shared use of personnel and equipment such as helicopters and rescue boats appropriate for medical emergencies.

Public safety agencies are most frequently the first responders to an emergency patient. The EMS system must therefore work with these agencies to ensure the use of special equipment, proper training of staff, linked communications, and the development of cooperative operating procedures.

8. *Consumer Participation*—The EMS system must make provisions in its system management that persons residing in the area and having no professional training or experience may participate in the policy making for the system.

While there is no federally required percentage of consumer participation in EMS planning or advisory organizations, reasonable consumer representation should be provided. One approach would be to involve the committee of the advisory council of the local CHP(b) Agency which has consumer representation. Any other advisory committee should include consumers who have access to the system administrators regarding plans and operations of the EMS system.

9. *Accessibility to Care*—The EMS system must provide necessary emergency services to all patients without prior inquiry as to the ability of the patient to pay.

The EMS system must not require evidence of the ability to pay prior to care for the services of ambulance, hospital or critical care units. The system should provide measures to monitor for restrictive measures that may eliminate any person or group of people from equal quality of services within the region.

10. *Transfer of Patients*—The EMS system shall provide for transfer of patients to facilities and programs which offer such followup care

and rehabilitation as is necessary to effect the maximum recovery of the patient.

The transfer of emergency patients from the emergency site to the emergency department, critical care unit, and to followup care and rehabilitation centers are all within the scope of a total EMS system. The components of training, transportation, recordkeeping and others all interrelate to this continuum of care.

11. *Standardized Patient Recordkeeping*—Each EMS regional system shall provide for a standardized patient recordkeeping system which shall cover the treatment of the patient from initial entry into the system through his discharge from it, and shall be consistent with patient records used in followup care and rehabilitation of the patient.

Each applicant for an award of funds under Sections 1203 and 1204 is required to provide for a standardized recordkeeping system. It is intended that information be collected for patients from initial entry into the system. Differing levels of data acquisition will be required for the general and specific patient groups. Consideration must be given to the patient's records during the pre-hospital phase and inclusion of such records in the patient's emergency department record.

The minimal patient records necessary for the EMS system are the dispatcher records, the ambulance records and the emergency department records. In order to fulfill requirements of evaluation and reports to Congress, certain information must be able to be derived from these records:

- Patient identification information: the records must be designed so that the dispatcher record, ambulance record and emergency department record on each patient can be compared for evaluation and management purposes.
- Patient access information: How did the patient access the system (arrive at emergency department)?
- Timing of ambulance services: response time, time at scene, and travel time to hospital.
- Patient condition: at scene, upon arrival in emergency department, and critical care unit.
- Patient treatment: at scene, during transport, in hospital.
- Patient diagnostic and treatment services: at emergency department, hospital and critical care unit.
- Disposition of patient: discharged, referred for out-patient care, referred to another hospital, admitted, died.

• Condition of patient: at discharge from emergency department, hospital and critical care unit.

Specific required minimum data elements which are to be included on the patient records will be described in a future publication "EMS Patient Record-Keeping System Handbook." Optional data elements will also be described in this publication. Advice will be given on the design and management of the data system. General management and specific impact evaluation programs required from each grantee should be developed as part of the grant application.

12. *Public Information and Education*—The EMS system shall provide programs of public education and information for all people in the area so they know about the system, how to access it, and how to use it properly.

The information program should take into account the needs of visitors to, as well as residents of, that area to know or be able to learn immediately the means of obtaining EMS. Programs should stress the general dissemination of information regarding appropriate methods of medical self-help and first-aid and the availability of first-aid training programs in the area.

An EMS system can have the best equipment, employ highly trained personnel and provide quality care, but if the people of the community do not understand: (1) What is an EMS system? (2) How can it help me? and (3) How do I use it?, the system is worthless. The purpose of the information and education component is to provide local citizens with an acceptable understanding about EMS and provide information on a periodic basis to local people.

13. *Independent Review and Evaluation*—Each EMS system must provide for (1) periodic, comprehensive, and independent review and evaluation of the extent and quality of the emergency health care services provided in the system's service area and (2) submission to the Secretary of the reports of each such review and evaluation.

Each grant recipient under Section 1203 and 1204 is required to submit as part of the final performance report, an independent review and evaluation of the regional EMS system. It is intended that such review and evaluation be periodic and comprehensive so that changes in emergency health care can be determined. The evaluation should be conducted by a qualified organization other than the grantee. The grant application should indicate plans for this evaluation or plans for selecting an evaluator.

There is no intention to require sophisticated and expensive research oriented evaluation from funds granted under Sections 1203 and 1204. What is required is that persons not associated with the project conduct a review and evaluation of the extent and quality of the services provided. As a minimum the reviewer should have available to him:

- A description of the EMS resources, capability and performance measures at the start of the period being evaluated.
- A description of the interventions brought about during the period to include clinical and EMS component elements.
- A description of the EMS resources, capability and performance measures at the end of the period being evaluated.
- The description of the achievements of performance measures of the EMS system referred to above. There should be at a minimum an analysis of 14 days performance throughout the year. The 14 days should be a modified random sample chosen so that there is at least one day for each month and two replications of each day of the week. Total numbers of calls for ambulance service and of emergency department patient visits should also be reported.
- The report should include a description of the system's resources, capability and performance and also analytical tables to reflect inventory changes, component activity and patient care services.
- Clinical output or impact evaluations of death and disability should include those clinical patient groups that have been specifically addressed in the operations application and include samples of the major categories. General patient population studies as well as specific patient group analysis will have local and national relevance.

14. *Disaster Linkage*—The EMS system must have a plan to assure that the system will be capable of providing emergency medical services in the system's service area during mass casualties, natural disasters or national emergencies.

The EMS system is not the regional health disaster organization. It is the emergency medical organization that will work with other agencies during a disaster to provide emergency medical care. The EMS system must be linked to the local, regional and State disaster plans and participate in exercises to test disaster plans.

15. *Mutual Aid Agreements*—Each EMS system must provide for the establishment of appropriate arrangements with EMS systems or similar entities serving neighboring areas for the provision of emergency medical services on a reciprocal basis where access to such services would be more appropriate and effective in terms of the services available, time and distance.

Arrangement among EMS regional systems and similar entities serving neighboring areas shall be written agreements, signed by individuals authorized to act for the respective parties with respect to such agreements, and reviewed and reevaluated at least once a year. Such agreements should cover the exchange of service coverage, communication linkages, licensure and certification, and reimbursement (as appropriate).

D. Evaluation of EMS as a Component of the Total Health Care Delivery System

A national EMS goal will be the assistance and guidance in the regional planning and operation of sound emergency medical care delivery programs. Significant lessons can be realized in the utilization of fixed and mobile facilities, the use of a wider spectrum of health care specialists, and the integration of this emergency health care effort with other ongoing public and private community service programs.

The coordination of established medical and safety efforts brings the emergency medical care program to an interface with community service activities heretofore outside the scope of established medical practice. Community involvement by a wide spectrum of the public, private, and governmental entities gives an emergency medical service system a new dimension to health care that has not previously been a major consideration in American medical practice.

An additional result of the regional EMS system effort will be the demonstration of how other essential non-emergent health services and programs might be stylized similar to EMS on a geographic and service demand basis. Some experience already suggests that programs such as blood, organ transplantation and rehabilitation as well as quality assurance programs might be enhanced by regional systems models. EMS planners and operations managers must become aware of the need to reexamine the mechanisms by which reimbursement can be provided through a systems approach. This approach will require a reexamination of economic and fiscal sources of coverage for services, and rates of reimbursement for direct payment, third party insurers, and public funds.

The National EMS System effort will improve the quality of care for critically injured and ill citizens across the country. Because of its unique characteristics, emergency medical care provides a rare opportunity for experience in many other phases of health care delivery. It is anticipated that the "ripple effect" in the EMS effort may extend beyond the limits of acute care phases into many functional component areas.

The success of any EMS system will be dependent upon the wisdom and appropriate integration of resources, operations management and financial planning into an effective program. The major task of the Division of Emergency Medical Services will be to provide current and timely technical assistance and guidance by use of the established and operational EMS Demonstration Projects.

E. EMS Systems Management

National experience with public and private funds has demonstrated that a few strategic factors are paramount to a successful EMS system effort.

The following components must be addressed in order to develop and integrate a total EMS system.

- Action Plan for EMSS Area—A comprehensive and detailed plan should be created for establishment, operation, and expansion of the EMS "care" system.
- *Lead Agency*—A lead agency should be identified as responsible for the EMS system including grants management control and operations coordination of the involved community and regional organizations.
- *Financial Support*—Appropriate means of financial support for initial and continued EMS operations must be considered. Such financial support may be derived from various Federal programs, State and local funds, general revenue sharing funds, third party payments and direct payments from patients.

The intent of the EMSS Act is to fund EMS projects on a multi-governmental and multi-community basis. At the present time there are a few regions in the country where an appropriate regional health authority exists. Such an organization or special health consortium may be developed or the applicant must rely on the established State health office with its management and regulatory capability.

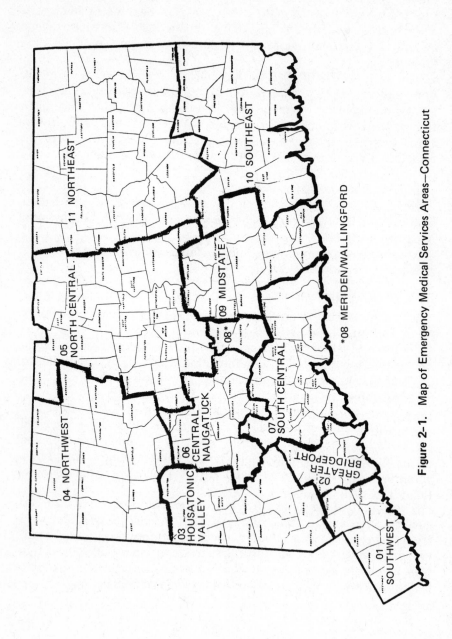

Figure 2-1. Map of Emergency Medical Services Areas—Connecticut

※ *Chapter 2*

Launching the Connecticut Study—
Plan and Methodology

EMS IN CONNECTICUT—1970

As we began our efforts in Connecticut in 1970, the state
of the art of emergency medical services was far more
rudimentary than it is today. As in most of the nation,
no well-planned or organized system for emergency care existed.

Aware that little had been done statewide in this field, and
through leadership provided by the Yale Trauma Program, a group of
concerned citizens formed an ad hoc committee on emergency medical services in December 1970 to begin to work toward improvements in EMS in the state. The committee's members served on a
voluntary basis because of their interest and commitment to the
field. The ad hoc committee grew and met monthly to address various aspects of emergency care.

In late 1971, at the request of the state health commissioner and
the governor's representative of the State Department of Transportation, the ad hoc committee was officially designated as the
Connecticut Advisory Committee on Emergency Medical Services,
and advised both departments in this field.[a] The Committee thus
assumed statewide leadership for emergency medical services.

[a] A list of the Advisory Committee members is included in Appendix 2A.

41

The first effort undertaken by the ad hoc committee was obtaining an allocation of $30,000 of U.S. Department of Transportation funds for the training of emergency medical technicians in early 1971. Until that time, no DOT funds had been used for EMS in Connecticut and, except for a pilot course at Norwalk Hospital, no EMTs had been trained in the state.

Recognizing the lack of requisite data for statewide EMS planning, the Committee placed top priority on conducting a comprehensive statewide study. In May 1971 the Yale Trauma Program was given the charge to carry out this activity under the supervision and direction of the EMS Advisory Committee.

The study analyzed: emergency ambulance services (Chapter 3), emergency medical communications (Chapter 4), costs of ambulance services (Chapter 5), hospital emergency departments (Chapter 6), emergency department physicians (Chapter 7), emergency department nurses and other ED personnel (Chapter 8) and legal and regulatory issues (Chapter 9). A statement of findings, recommendations, and priorities appears in Chapter 10. The epilogue (Chapter 11) reviews important events since the submission of the completed study to Governor Thomas J. Meskill in December 1972.

INPUT, PROCESS, AND OUTCOME

An ideal study of EMS would measure input (resources related to patient needs), process (actual use of services), and outcome (the outcome of a patient's condition.[1] Since outcome is a function of resources, the patient's clinical condition, and service utilization (input plus process), criteria should be selected that, ideally, measure the separate effect on outcome of different levels of input and resource utilization. Mortality rates are not a sufficient outcome measure because they are often insensitive to change or are affected only slightly by changes in EMS subelements. Another significant problem in outcome measurement is that the outcome of one subsystem becomes an input for another subsystem. For example, any study of the effectiveness of emergency department care must consider and control for the level of care provided prior to the patient's arrival in the emergency department.

Accordingly, it is doubtful that one set of outcomes for the entire EMS system is possible. Rather, a sequential set of input-process-outcome-input data from a series of subsystems is preferred. Gibson suggests some valid measures of outcome but warns that a sufficiently large data base for each clinical condition and each EMS element will be necessary to consider the effect of clinical severity and to evaluate individual EMS elements.[2]

Until the needed outcome measures are developed and validated, EMS studies will have to rely on utilization measures and such structural elements as personnel, facilities, equipment, organization, and costs. This is the approach we selected.

NEED VS. DEMAND

An ideal EMS study would also distinguish between a population's need for EMS and its demand. Demand is only some portion of the total need and while demand is measurable and finite, need is ill-defined and difficult to quantify. An inventory of need would identify the medical conditions, ailments, and handicaps of all potential EMS users, translate these conditions into EMS requirements for EMS, and relate this information to social, demographic and geographic characteristics of the population.

Demand can be measured by determining the frequency of requests for various kinds of services. However, this measure is insensitive to the effects of differences in accessibility to these services and to questions of the necessity for a particular service such as whether the services rendered were medically required. The insensitivity of demand measures to access factors is a serious shortcoming and a principal reason why demand is often not an accurate indicator of need. Demand identifies only those individuals who manage to enter the EMS system. Those who do not know how to enter the system or who find access too costly or complex are omitted from demand analysis.

To complicate matters further, gross demand data include EMS use by patients not requiring emergency treatment, which might be considered illegitimate or inefficient use of EMS resources. Thus, demand measures usually tend to overestimate the legitimate use of EMS resources but underestimate the actual need for EMS.[3] We attempted a detailed analysis of need and demand in one area of the state but because of the constraints mentioned above, it was of such limited value to the overall analysis that it will not be presented here.

STEPS IN CARRYING OUT THE STUDY

Step 1: Developing Study Goals

As the individuals responsible for undertaking the study, our first task was to establish clear-cut goals. We believed that these goals should not be established by the research team alone but in conjunction with those responsible for implementing and operating the EMS system. Without such input, no study is likely to have maximum impact. Therefore, we worked with the elected representatives of commercial and volunteer ambulance associations, with representatives from hospital emergency departments (administrators, physicians, and nurses), police departments, fire departments, and appropriate local elected officials. The formation of a representative and working advisory committee was crucial to this effort.

Working in cooperation with the EMS Advisory Committee, we established the following study goals:

1. Identify the strengths and deficiencies in the emergency-care system in Connecticut
2. Make recommendations necessary to remedy these deficiencies
3. Set priorities, identify agencies, and establish a schedule to implement the recommendations.

Step 2: Defining the Study Population

Because Connecticut is a small state and contains a diversity (size, type, geographical distribution) of EMS services, we felt it was both desirable and feasible to seek a 100 percent sample of EMS providers. Another advantage of seeking a 100 percent sample and participation of all providers is the higher likelihood for successful implementation of study findings.

Accordingly, we attempted to collect and analyze data from the emergency departments of all 35 acute general hospitals, the 179 ambulance services based in 169 towns, the 324 fire departments; the 89 local police departments, the 11 state police barracks, and the 49 resident state troopers providing police and EMS service to 49 towns; and all emergency department physicians, nurses, and allied health personnel. While the original goal of a 100 percent sample of all EMS resources and services was not attained, the study sample included a good representation of EMS providers in terms of geographical distribution, public-private mix, and volume of services rendered (see Table 2-1).

Step 3: Data-Collection Period

The study period chosen was July 1 to November 1, 1971. Manpower, costs, and time constraints precluded a longer data-collection period. Although the time chosen does not include seasonal variations and holidays, it does cover high-volume months resulting from summer travel. This higher demand period may skew the data slightly, but it has the advantage of permitting planning for peak

Table 2-1. EMS Providers in Connecticut Study

Type of Provider	Number in Connecticut	Number in Study	Percent in Study
Hospital emergency departments	35	35	100
Ambulance services	166[a]	141[a]	85
Fire departments	324	168	54
Local police departments	89	72	81
State police barracks	11	11	100
Resident state police troopers	49	40	85
ED physicians	224	109	49
ED nurses (RNs)	359	256	71
ED nurses (LPNs)	52	30	58
ED aides/orderlies	93	62	67
Other ED technicians	15	10	67
Emergency medical technicians[b]	211	109	52

[a]Thirteen additional special services were excluded because they provided service only to limited population groups.

[b]This was the group that took the first series of six EMT courses given in Connecticut.

times. Figure 2–1 displays the time consumed by all components of the study. If time, manpower, and funds permitted, a longer prospective study would have been preferable. We advocate the prospective method where possible because in our experience the data necessary for EMS planning are often not recorded routinely and accurately.

Step 4: Study Design and Data Collection

We began by undertaking an exhaustive review and analysis of existing EMS literature, including other statewide studies. Comprehensive interview documents for hospitals and ambulance services were prepared. Additional interview documents and questionnaires were developed to focus on specific EMS elements such as ED physicians and nurses, EMTs, police and fire departments (regarding communications), and hospital ED costs. These were developed during five eight-hour sessions with the full study team and many other meetings including discussions with members of the Advisory Committee and faculty colleagues. Personal interviews were utilized whenever feasible, with mailed questionnaires used only when interviews were not possible. Where possible, the survey instrument utilized closed responses but some open-ended questions were required. The instruments were designed on a branching basis so that questions regarding a specific component of EMS could be asked of appropriate individuals.

We directed and supervised the interview team, which was composed of nine MPH candidates in the Yale Hospital Administration

Project Activities	1971						1972												1973	
	July	Aug.	Sept.	Oct.	Nov.	Dec.	Jan.	Feb.	Mar.	Apr.	May	June	July	Aug.	Sept.	Oct.	Nov.	Dec.	Jan.	Feb.
Planning for data collection	▮	▮																		
Data collection		▮	▮	▮																
Description and analysis of current EMS			▮	▮	▮	▮	▮	▮												
Identification of deficiencies in EMS						▮	▮	▮												
Development of recommendations								▮	▮	▮	▮	▮	▮	▮	▮	▮				
Development of a phased plan of implementation										▮	▮	▮	▮	▮	▮	▮				
Submission of report to Governor and Department of Transportation																		▮		
Preparation and dissemination of blueprint for change																			▮	

Figure 2–1. Schedule of Activities for Connecticut EMS Study

Program. Their knowledge of the subject and of research methods shortened the design phase.

For the purposes of data collection, the state was divided into nine regions, each containing approximately equal numbers of hospitals, ambulance services, fire and police departments, and population. Each member of the interview team was assigned a region in which to interview the appropriate personnel. In the case of hospitals, the administrator, an assistant, the comptroller, the chief of nursing, the head emergency department nurse, and the physician in charge of the ED were interviewed.

Prior to actual data collection, each team member pretested the interview instruments with appropriate EMS individuals. The instrument was then revised, and interpretation of each question was agreed upon by the study team at team meetings.

Interviewing sessions consumed considerable time. Hospital interviews required the equivalent of a one-day visit. Depending on availability of personnel, some interviews were spread over several days or even weeks. Interviews were conducted at thirty-one hospitals. At the remaining four institutions, questionnaires were mailed to staff personnel, and these were later reviewed with hospital officials to ensure completeness of information and accuracy of interpretation.

Step 5: Enhancing Participation in the Study

To enhance the response rate to the survey instruments, potential participants were briefed by the study directors, and letters of support were sent by officials of state associations and agencies. Although time-consuming, the importance of personal meetings with official representatives and members of the private and volunteer ambulance associations, the Commissioner of Health, the Connecticut Hospital Association, the Connecticut Medical Society, and the state chapter of the American College of Emergency Physicians proved valuable. At these meetings, the purpose of the study was reviewed, and often valuable input regarding the survey instrument was obtained. When followed with official letters of introduction, appointments for data collection were usually not difficult to obtain, and cooperation was enhanced. Members of the EMS Advisory Committee were particularly helpful in this important step.

Step 6: Data Analysis

Data were grouped and analyzed according to widely used statistical measures. Frequency distributions and measures of central tendency (mean, median, and mode) were most commonly used. Where appropriate, more sophisticated analytical techniques such as linear regression and statistical tests of significance were applied. The majority of EMS services were evaluated by comparing them with guidelines of professional organizations, e.g., the American College of Surgeons, the National Academy of Sciences, the U.S. Department of Transportation, and the Joint Commission on Accreditation of Hospitals. We believe that these guidelines were the most comprehensive and valid at the time of the study.

Step 7: Preparing the Report

Upon completion of data analysis, a draft report was prepared and distributed to the EMS Advisory Committee. Findings and recommendations were discussed by the study team and the Committee at several lengthy meetings, with suggestions incorporated into the final report. Various aspects of the study were presented in draft form at meetings with representatives of the state medical society, the state hospital association, comprehensive health planning directors, the volunteer and commercial ambulance associations, the fire and police chiefs' associations, the state nurses' association, and the state regional medical program, among others. These meetings were important in explaining details of the report and in gaining the support of interested EMS groups. The final report, incorporating suggestions from these interested parties, was submitted to the governor and the U.S. Department of Transportation on December 15, 1972[4] (see Chapter 10).

Step 8: Implementing the Findings

Upon completion of the report, the EMS Advisory Committee and members of the study team worked to implement the study findings. Recognizing that the detailed 700-page report would not receive wide readership, we prepared a 52-page summary booklet entitled *Emergency Medical Services in Connecticut: A Blueprint for Change*[5] to enhance understanding of the study's recommendations. *A Blueprint for Change* was distributed widely throughout the state and gave its readers ready familiarity with the state's EMS problems and priorities. Most important, it spelled out the study's findings and priorities in summary form for the governor and state legislators, the individuals ultimately responsible for enacting the legislation necessary to reform EMS in Connecticut. The blueprint was sent to all elected state officials, to community leaders, and to many interested groups (see Chapter 11). Informal meetings with members of the state legislature and the governor's staff were held. Concerned Connecticut citizens, Advisory Committee members, and the study team performed this function together.

SPECIFIC METHODOLOGIES UTILIZED

The collection of data on various EMS components required a number of specially tailored approaches. In addition to the general steps outlined above, the following methodologies were used to collect data on ambulance services, manpower, and communications. (The approaches used in studying the cost and legislative issues are discussed in Chapters 5 and 9.)

Ambulance Services

Data regarding demographic characteristics, gross health statistics, projected population figures, projected land-use patterns, and projected traffic patterns were available from state and local governmental agencies.

Prospective data regarding ambulance use were obtained through responses to four typewritten pages of questions covering important aspects of each call for ambulance service. This questionnaire was completed for every call received during a one-week period (Aug. 27–Sept. 5, 1971) for commercial purveyors and a two-week period (Aug. 23–Sept. 5, 1971) for all other ambulance purveyors. Approximately 65 percent of all ambulance services responded by submitting completed forms for calls during the designated period (assuming complete reporting).

The short periods were a result of the purveyors' understandable reluctance to participate for a longer time. One week was chosen for commercial purveyors because of their large volume of calls, while a two-week period was necessary for other ambulance purveyors, which had smaller call volumes (see Chapter 3).

A somewhat crude but simple check of validity and reliability was undertaken by quantifying the degree of similarity between the prospective and retrospective call samples. Annual ambulance-call volume was estimated from the actual volume for each purveyor recorded during the prospective study and was then matched with the estimate expressed by the same purveyor in the retrospective study ambulance interview document. Of the ambulance services that estimated their annual call volume retrospectively, eighty-three participated in prospective data collection.

Each set of estimates was investigated by means of correlation analysis. A sample, consisting of matched pairs of call volumes from prospective and restrospective samples, was constructed and used to assess the internal consistency of study data. The results were encouraging in that the estimates from both samples were comparable.

In the first comparison, we grouped paired calls estimated by type of purveyor (commercial, municipal, and volunteer). Correlation analyses were then conducted separately for each major purveyor group. Consistency between estimates was best for municipal emergency ambulance services (EAS), which demonstrated a high correlation (coefficient, $r = 0.91$). Perfect correspondence between estimates would be indicated by $r = 1.00$, with $r = 0.7$ and above considered acceptable. Analysis of thirty-seven volunteer services also showed a high correlation ($r = 0.85$). The poorest correlation was found in the analysis of estimates for sixteen commercial ambulance services ($r = 0.74$). Sample sizes and correlation coefficients are shown in Table 2-2.

The same type of analysis was performed on the data grouped by health service region (see Table 2-2). Most correlations were in the high ranges of 0.88 and above. For reasons we could not determine, an atypically low correlation coefficient ($r = 0.57$) was obtained for the Bridgeport region. Insufficient information (i.e., only one paired data observation) was available for the Waterbury region.

Table 2-2. Prospective and Retrospective Call Samples by Health Service Region and by Type of Ambulance Purveyor

Health Service Region	Number of EAS Purveyors Responding	Correlation Coefficient
Bridgeport	5	.57
Capital	24	.88
Danbury	6	.96[a]
Middletown	5	.98
Northeast	7	.83[a]
Northwest	7	.98[a]
South Central	8	.95
Southeast	8	.88[a]
Southwest	12	.99
Waterbury	1	—

Type of Purveyor		
Commercial	16	.74
Municipal	30	.91
Volunteer	37	.85

[a]Includes no commercial ambulance data.

It would be useful to generalize that, from a methodological standpoint, retrospective utilization data, even though estimated in many cases, are as accurate as the more costly and time-consuming prospective data. While this may be so—and, indeed, the relationship appears fairly strong in this study's results—caution must be used in making predictions from a data base that in other cases may be relatively soft. One way to circumvent the costly prospective technique is to undertake sample prospective studies, like the one described above, and compare the results with retrospective estimates.

Because of the variety of organizational forms involved in ambulance services, a typology of definitions is useful. We used two typologies—one for general study purposes (see Chapter 3) and the other designed especially for cost analysis (see Chapter 5).

Identification of existing ambulance services proved difficult, despite a 1970 questionnaire survey issued by the Connecticut State Health Department which identified 160 ambulance services. The department had no information concerning the location or number of services established since the 1970 survey or concerning ambulance services that had ceased operation in the intervening year. Because we wished to contact all of Connecticut's emergency ambulance services, we resurveyed the state.

The department's listing was updated by incorporating information provided in interviews with hospital personnel, searching through telephone books, and calling police and fire departments. The ambulance purveyors cooperated by providing knowledge of other services, and the interview team investigated these leads. As a result of these efforts, 179 emergency ambulance services were identified as providing service to the public.[b]

For the purpose of data collection each interviewer was assigned an EMS study area that included approximately twenty ambulance services. Each member of the investigating team scheduled the interviews with the ambulance services in the assigned area. Prior to the interviews, letters were sent to commercial purveyors from the Connecticut Ambulance Association and to municipal and volunteer purveyors from the Connecticut Volunteer Ambulance Association explaining the purpose and scope of the study. A personal visit was made to the director or designated representative of each ambulance service. In a few instances, because ambulance purveyors were not

[b]Several services in New York, Massachusetts, and Rhode Island cover border areas of Connecticut. These were not interviewed directly but were included in some of the Connecticut responses regarding backup vehicles and interservice communications.

immediately available for personal interview, questionnaires were mailed to them and followed by personal interviews.

To identify, define, and describe ambulance services, a descriptive analysis of selected variables for three categories—commercial, volunteer, and municipal—was undertaken. Two descriptive analytical techniques were applied to the data—percentage determinations of selected variables as well as simple counts of the numbers of cases of selected variables in each of the three categories. The ability of commercial, volunteer, and municipal ambulance services to meet the nine funding criteria used by the National Highway Traffic Safety Administration of the U.S. Department of Transportation was assessed by applying appropriate chi-square tests (see Chapter 3). (Selection of the chi-square test was dependent upon the nature and type of data collected.)

Emergency Department Physicians

Physicians eligible for inclusion in the study were selected on the basis of the physician-hospital relationship. Because the hospital-salaried arrangement implied physician commitment to EMS, method of payment was used to determine the study population. Both full-time hospital-based EMS physicians and part-time nonhospital-based EMS physicians were included. Though the implied degree of commitment to EMS was less with the latter group, it was included because the part-time pattern was the most common hospital-paid physician staffing arrangement (see Chapter 7).

Names and mailing addresses of physicians were compiled through use of the section on staffing in the hospital interview instrument. In the course of conducting the hospital visits, we instructed the members of our research team to give a brief description of the entire project and request a mailing list for all the full- and part-time EMS physicians. By the end of the data collection, twenty-six of the twenty-eight hospitals with hospital-paid physician coverage complied with this request.

The mailing lists from the twenty-six cooperating hospitals contained names and addresses of 215 physicians. To this were added the names and addresses of 9 hospital-paid EMS physicians from a list provided by the American College of Emergency Physicians (ACEP). The survey sample of 224 physicians represented 78 percent of the 289 physicians identified by the hospital questionnaire as being full- or part-time hospital-salaried physicians.

Questionnaires were mailed to the 224 physicians with a covering letter of explanation and a stamped, self-addressed envelope. After an encouraging initial response, a second letter was mailed to nonrespondents reiterating the objectives of the survey and soliciting cooperation.

Of the 224 questionnaires mailed, 109 were returned and considered appropriate for analysis. The number of physicians in the study sample represented 49 percent of the total study population. Sixty-six percent of full-time EMS physicians responded in contrast to 22 percent of part-time EMS physicians.

Emergency Department Nurses and Other ED Personnel

Our objectives for this part of the study were to identify and describe (1) nonphysician personnel within hospital EDs, (2) nonphysician staffing patterns employed by hospitals to satisfy ED work load, and (3) emergency medical technicians (EMTs) recently trained throughout the state.[c] Individual questionnaires were prepared for each of five categories: registered nurses, licensed practical nurses, aides/orderlies, other emergency-care personnel, and emergency medical technicians. A questionnaire on staffing patterns, completed by directors of nursing in the thirty-five short-term hospitals, was also developed.

Pilot interviews were the first step in the development of these questionnaires, using as respondents personnel employed in the emergency department of Yale-New Haven Hospital. Appointments were made with each of the inhospital professionals to discuss the type of information desired, the proper wording of questions, and the types of responses to be used for checklist answers. Pilot interviews for the EMT data instrument were arranged with recent graduates of the EMT course employed by an ambulance service in New Haven.

Personnel in each category were asked questions which fit into the following two groups:

1. Quantitative descriptors
   a. Employment status
   b. Age, sex, race

[c]We conducted a separate study of the first group of 201 EMTs trained in Connecticut in 1971 to develop a profile of the graduates, obtain their assessment of the EMT course, and to understand their role in EMS. Their response was valuable in confirming the effectiveness of and need for such training. These data will not be presented here because of the small size of the study population in relation to the total number of EMTs now trained in Connecticut (over 4,000), and because of the preliminary nature of the findings. G. Starr, "A Description and Analysis of Non-Physician Manpower in Emergency Medical Services in Connecticut," master's thesis, Department of Epidemiology and Public Health, Yale University School of Medicine, New Haven, Connecticut, 1972.

    c. Salary/wage levels
    d. Educational background
    e. Experience in nursing and EMS
    f. Training for nursing and EMS
    g. Other job specialties
2. Qualitative descriptors
    a. Preference for EMS work
    b. Most desirable and least desirable aspects of EMS
    c. Opportunities to advance in skills and knowledge (asked of aide/orderlies and other technicians only)
    d. Willingness to take further training under certain conditions (e.g., paid off-duty time)
    e. Capability of performing more responsible tasks

Underlying our design of the qualitative questions were two premises: that certain groups of personnel were not being utilized as fully as would be possible if given adequate training and opportunity and that special job-preference factors were responsible for the choice of EMS work over other areas in the hospital. Open-ended questions directed the respondents to indicate in their own words the tasks they could perform or the conditions they considered most or least desirable. Closed-response or checklist answers were avoided because of the possibility of bias and because the development of more sophisticated attitude measurements such as Likert scales was not possible within the time span of the study.

Task lists, attached to the personnel questionnaires given to all but the EMTs, were developed after the pretest of the basic questionnaires. The *Uniform Manpower Evaluation Protocol* was a major source for identifying forty-three tasks generally performed in hospital emergency departments.[7] The task list was designed to elicit information indicating which functions various professional levels of personnel now perform as well as which they feel they could, should, or should not perform.

As a realistic base upon which to draw inferences from the nonphysicians' responses to forty-three tasks, a similar task list was proposed for physicians employed in emergency departments. The physician task list was essentially the same as the nonphysician questionnaire, but it included some additional tasks. Its content was discussed with the chairman of the Connecticut chapter of the ACEP to clarify the document's intent and purpose. Physicians were asked to indicate the "lowest" professional category that could be expected to perform each task (with the assumption that the professional had been properly trained) under two separate conditions:

with and without a physician present. Thus, there were two possible responses in each task. Also, a "physician only" response was provided for tasks that the physicians felt should not be delegated. This task list for physicians was distributed along with the mailed questionnaires discussed earlier.

The intent of this task list was to develop a basis for a group of tasks that could be incorporated into expanded job roles for nonphysician personnel in emergency departments. Both nonphysician and physician input was thought to be desirable (see Chapter 8).

An additional staffing-pattern questionnaire was sent to the directors of nursing of each hospital to clarify variations in the responses to the original EMS staffing interviews and to provide more complete staffing information. Before distribution, the document was discussed with a member of the nursing administration at Yale-New Haven Hospital to clarify its purpose and content. The questionnaire sought information on scheduled man-hours for three eight-hour shifts per day by professional category. Four personnel categories were included: RN, LPN, aide/orderly, and other. The staffing-pattern data were obtained to complement the overall description of emergency medical personnel by pointing out the differences or similarities in institutional policies toward employing nonphysicians.

We found linear-regression techniques to be useful in studying alternative manpower mixes. While they do not purport to develop "correct" staffing for an emergency department based on an expected number of visits, they can show in quantitative and graphic terms how hospitals provide for staffing based on patient-visit statistics.

Emergency Medical Communications

We used two data-collection techniques to gather information related to emergency medical communications. One was the interview survey form developed for hospitals and ambulance services described earlier. The other was a mailed questionnaire for police and fire departments designed to obtain essential information about emergency-call reception and response activities.

As mentioned earlier, the response rates from Connecticut hospitals, ambulance companies, state police, and local police departments and fire departments were exceptionally good (see Table 2-1). We attribute this to the measures taken in Step 5 and to the covering letters accompanying questionnaires from the state hospital association, state police commissioner, commercial and volunteer ambulance associations, Connecticut Police Chiefs Association, and the state fire coordinator.

Having presented the various methodologies utilized, we now turn to a presentation of our data and findings.

Appendix 2A

Connecticut Advisory Committee on Emergency Medical Services (1972)

Mr. Robert Bergeron, Director of Education, Connecticut Hospital Association

Mr. Todd Berman, Associate Director, Connecticut Hospital Planning Commission

Mr. George Booth, Assistant Administrator, Park City Hospital

Mr. Norman Booth, Associate Highway Engineer, Bureau of Highways

Mr. Thomas Brask, Director of Communications, Yale Trauma Program

Mr. Edward A. Carroll, Chief, Engineering Division, Motor Vehicle Department

Dr. John Christoforo, Director, Emergency Department, Hospital of St. Raphael

Mr. Joseph Finnegan, President, Connecticut Volunteer Ambulance Association

Mr. Laurence M. Ford, Fire Coordinator, Connecticut Civil Defense

Mr. Marshall Frankel, Chief, Disaster Health Services Division, Conn. State Health Department

Lt. Michael Griffin, Connecticut State Police

Dr. Elliot M. Gross, Chief Medical Examiner, State of Connecticut

Dr. Robert Huszar, Director of Research, St. Francis Hospital

Dr. Ernest Izumi, Laboratory Director, New Milford Hospital

Dr. Kristaps J. Keggi, Chairman, Committee on Trauma, Connecticut Chapter, American College of Surgeons

Mr. Paul Lally, Coordinator, Emergency Department, Yale-New Haven Hospital

Mr. Joseph Lansing, Bridgeport Ambulance Service

Mr. Guy McKinstry, Assistant Administrator, Stamford Hospital

Dr. Charles Parton, Director, Emergency Department, Hartford Hospital

Dr. Richard Pepler, Dunlap and Associates, Inc.

Mr. John Post, Dean of Academic Affairs, Post Junior College

Dr. Joseph Reese, New Milford Hospital

Dr. Edward A. Rem, Director, Emergency Department, Norwalk Hospital

Dr. Alfred M. Sadler, Jr., Director, Yale Trauma Program (Chairman)

Mr. Blair L. Sadler, Co-Director, Yale Trauma Program

Mr. John Sullivan, Director of Continuing Education, Post Junior College

Ms. Carol von Stein, Yale Trauma Program

Dr. Samuel B. Webb Jr., Associate Professor of Public Health, Department of Epidemiology and Public Health, Yale University School of Medicine

Part II

The Pre-Hospital Phase

✳ *Chapter 3*

Emergency Ambulance Services

INTRODUCTION AND OBJECTIVES

For much of the past quarter of a century, ambulances have been used primarily for transporting the sick and injured quickly to a hospital where definitive care could begin. This was not always the case. Originally developed during the Napoleonic wars, the ambulance was designed to serve as a mobile hospital.[1] While generally not accepted in the United States today, the mobile hospital concept is still alive in parts of Western Europe and has recently been resurrected in this country with the advent of specialized units for the care of heart-disease patients.[2,3]

Historical differences notwithstanding, it is generally agreed that ambulance vehicles must be properly constructed and adequately equipped, must respond rapidly to calls for assistance, and must be staffed for administering emergency medical care on site and en route to the hospital. Such services should be organized so that a patient is taken to the hospital emergency facility best equipped to render the particular care needed (see Chapter 6). Unfortunately, emergency ambulance services (EAS) fall far short of these minimal characteristics in many areas of the United States.[4]

This chapter presents selected findings regarding an evaluation of Connecticut's ambulance services. We examined seven important components of ambulance services:

1. Emergency service coverage
2. Personnel

3. Vehicles and equipment
4. Organization
5. Operational policies
6. Performance times
7. Evaluation criteria

In October 1971, our survey identified 179 emergency ambulance services of four major organizational types: commercial, volunteer, municipal, and special. The number of each that were identified and interviewed are shown in Table 3-1. For the purposes of this study, an emergency ambulance service by definition is one that provides care at the emergency scene and transports the patient to a hospital when needed. Because the "special" ambulance organizations mentioned in Chapter 2 were found to service a select and very limited population (e.g., industry, race tracks, or parks), attention was directed to the 141 of the 166 commercial, volunteer, and municipal services that participated in the study. (See Chapter 2 for the methodology employed.)

EMERGENCY SERVICE COVERAGE

Most Connecticut residents (92 percent) are provided with emergency ambulance services by organizations located within their own town limits. Volunteer services are most widely distributed, and in the densely populated southwest part of the state and the moderately populated southeast, volunteer organizations provide service to small geographic areas, usually their own towns. In the rural parts of the state, volunteers service larger geographic areas. Municipal ambulances are similar to volunteer ambulances in distribution, while commercial services are located primarily in densely populated towns and cover large geographic areas.

While every Connecticut town is included in the emergency service area of at least one ambulance purveyor, overlapping areas exist in

Table 3-1. Ambulance Purveyors by Type and Number

Type	Identified		Interviewed	
	Number	Precent	Number	Percent
Commercial	34	20	30	21
Volunteer	78	47	63	45
Municipal	54	33	48	34
Total	166	100	141	100

about half the towns, resulting in duplication of service. The 141 respondent ambulance services provide emergency coverage to a total area twice the size of the state.

Of the commercial purveyors, 73 percent operate in an emergency service area with four or more other services. In contrast, 50 of Connecticut's 169 towns have only one emergency vehicle available twenty-four hours per day. The majority of these towns are rural and sparsely populated. Despite a general overlap of emergency service areas and availability of vehicles, 17 percent of the ambulance purveyors have no backup capability in their areas. Organizations without backup service include ten commercial, seven volunteer, and seven municipal services.

In Connecticut, the smaller the population, the greater the number of emergency vehicles available for that population. The range is from seven vehicles per 100,000 people for densely populated areas to twenty-three vehicles per 100,000 for sparsely populated areas. This is explained by the difficult terrain, poor access roads, and the isolated nature of rural areas. Hampered by such obstacles, many small rural towns have developed their own service rather than linking up to a larger service, even in the face of limited backup capability.

Services provided by ambulance purveyors can be grouped into three categories: (1) emergency treatment at the scene without transport (rescue service), (2) emergency transportation with or without treatment en route (emergency ambulance service), and (3) nonurgent transportation of patients on a scheduled basis (nonemergency ambulance service). While most Connecticut ambulance services offer a combination of these, emergency ambulance services by our definition must include transport and cannot limit their work to scheduled transfer cases.

In Connecticut, most ambulance organizations respond to all types of emergency calls. Two commercial purveyors do not respond to traffic accidents and transfer traffic-related calls to a municipal police department. Of the 141 services interviewed, 16 percent do not transport patients with psychiatric emergencies.

A breakdown by type of call is presented in Figure 3-1 (the data are adjusted for the 3,131 call volume obtained prospectively). Traffic-related emergencies represent approximately 19 percent of all emergencies and 13 percent of all ambulance calls according to the prospective data. Traffic-related EAS calls were a larger proportion of all ambulance emergencies in the rural regions (22 percent) than in the urban corridor regions (15 percent).

An analysis of prospective and retrospective call data by type and distribution suggests that emergency calls represent about two-thirds

All Ambulance Calls

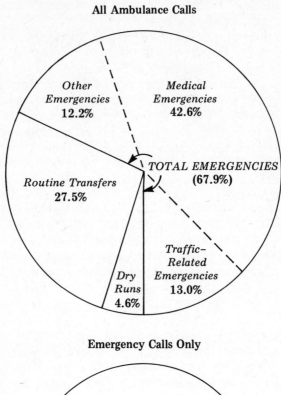

Emergency Calls Only

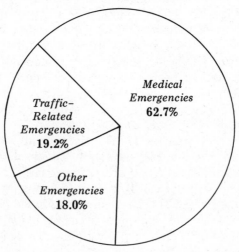

Figure 3–1. Percentage Breakdown of Ambulance Calls by Type of Call

of the state's ambulance calls. Dry runs comprise 4.6 percent of all emergency ambulance calls in the prospective study. (Dry runs include ambulance responses which require no medical care or transportation.) They represent larger percentages of all calls for municipal (6.1 percent) and volunteer (5.6 percent) services than for commercial units (3.5 percent). In addition to regular service coverage, forty-nine purveyors (thirteen commercial, nineteen volunteer, and seventeen municipal) provide special contractual or standby services. Standby services are used at sporting events, race tracks, industrial plants, beaches, and other large group functions. Because more and larger hospitals are located in urban corridor regions, these areas have a larger proportion of transfer cases (16 percent) than rural regions (10 percent).

We estimate that almost 66,000 emergency ambulance calls are received annually in Connecticut (see Appendix 3A). At the current rate of demand, this represents one ambulance call per day per 10,925 persons or a total ambulance call volume of 101,535 ambulance calls per year. More than 63 percent of Connecticut towns are estimated to receive, on the average, less than one ambulance call per day.

The inadequate record-keeping of Connecticut ambulance purveyors makes it difficult to determine annual call frequencies, much less mean increases on a yearly basis. Only 55 percent ($n = 78$) of the purveyors were able to report total emergency calls for the three-year period 1968–70. While generalizations are therefore suspect, the available data reveal some interesting facts.

On the average, there are about 390 emergency calls per year per ambulance service. While the commercial services constitute only one-sixth of the respondent purveyors, they performed almost 40 percent of all ambulance runs reported in 1970. The commercial services had about twice as many annual emergency calls as municipal operators and five times as many as volunteer services.

The volume of emergency calls among purveyors differs widely— in 1970, sixteen (21 percent) made fewer than 50 trips (and six of them made fewer than 25 trips), 42 percent made between 51 and 250 trips, and 37 percent made more than 250 trips annually. With a few exceptions, emergency ambulance operations are of modest scale, and most ambulance services in the state are utilized infrequently. Not surprisingly, our data reveal that the annual volume of emergency calls tends to be directly proportional to the population size of a given service area—i.e., the larger the population, the larger the volume of emergency calls.

In planning for adequate distribution of emergency ambulance services, some measure of the increase in volume of emergency calls over several years is necessary. As stated earlier, survey results on the mean increase in annual volume of emergency calls (1968–70) for the major purveyor groups were sketchy: only thirty-nine ambulance services (28 percent) provided the necessary information. From these limited data, it appears that the volume of emergency ambulance runs in Connecticut is growing at an annual rate of 10 to 15 percent.

The prospective study data indicate that for all but two hospitals most ambulance cases come from towns within the hospital's health service region as defined by the State Health Department. Only the emergency departments located in the Middletown and Danbury regions extend their service areas significantly into another region.

According to the prospective study, total calls for all purveyors are distributed evenly over the days of the week. However, traffic-related calls demonstrate a peaked distribution, with 53 percent occurring during the weekend (Friday through Sunday). Traffic-related calls represent about 20 percent of all EAS calls on Saturdays (compared to a daily average of 13 percent). More than two-thirds of all ambulance arrivals at Connecticut hospitals occur between 10:00 A.M. and 10:00 P.M.

All ambulance services provide twenty-four-hour coverage, either by personnel on the premises, standby personnel, or a combination of the two. Approximately 38 percent have driver/attendants on the premises, while 52 percent utilize standby personnel only. The latter is most common among the volunteer services. The remaining 10 percent have driver/attendants on the premises during the day and utilize standby coverage at night.

PERSONNEL

Approximately 27 percent of the emergency ambulance purveyors interviewed have no specific selection standards for driver/attendants. The majority of services require minimum standards regarding age, education, driving record, physical condition, lack of police record (no convictions for felonies or misdemeanors), and/or pre-employment medical training. Selection standards most frequently used for driver/attendants include:

1. Age—minimum age of eighteen years required by twenty-six purveyors (25 percent); minimum of twenty-one years required by sixty-five purveyors (63 percent)

2. Good driving records—required by 92 percent
3. No serious police record—required by 92 percent
4. Medical examination—required by 71 percent
5. Education—high school diploma required by 30 percent (primarily police and fire departments, which stipulate this for all employees).

Only 22 percent of Connecticut ambulance services require a minimum of an advanced Red Cross certificate before employing a driver-attendant. Preemployment training in the techniques of rescue and extrication procedures is rare. However, some type of first-aid training within thirty to sixty days after employment is required by 79 percent of the ambulance services. Of the 104 respondent services that require first-aid training, 69 percent require the standard Red Cross certificate, 71 percent require an Advanced Red Cross certificate, 3 percent require Emergency Medical Technician I (EMT I) training, 3 percent require the National Ambulance Training Institute (NATI) course, and 10 percent require some training in rescue equipment use and extrication procedures. These standards have risen significantly since 1971 with the administration of the eighty-one-hour EMT I course throughout the state (see Chapter 11).

Our survey attempted to determine the number of ambulance driver/attendants who had taken first-aid and rescue training courses during the two prior years (1969-71). Few purveyors could provide this information, but some tentative conclusions are possible. First, at the time of the 1971 study, the majority of driver/attendants enrolled in training courses received Red Cross instruction. Second, the majority of services requested that training courses be offered near towns in which their employees live so that interested parties can easily attend. Third, the EMT I training programs introduced in 1971 were well received.

It was encouraging to learn that fifty-three of the fifty-five emergency services with driver/attendants trained as EMTs in 1971 intend to continue sending personnel through this training program. Of the few services electing not to participate in the EMT course, the reasons cited were lack of money, problems of volunteers getting time off from regular jobs, and the feeling that EMT I training was unnecessary. (Advanced Red Cross training was considered sufficient.)

In addition to formal courses of instruction, in-service training can be an important element in maintaining competence. This is particularly true for volunteer purveyors, who often maintain a large number of personnel but manage few emergency calls annually. Only 25 percent of all purveyors hold regular in-service training programs. The incidence and frequency of in-service training among the three types of purveyors varies. Of the sixty volunteer services, 85 percent give in-service training, and 57 percent do so at least once a month. Of the forty-four municipal purveyors, 69 percent provide some in-service training, and 55 percent hold sessions at least once a month. Among the commercial purveyors, 57 percent give in-service training at least once a month, but 36 percent provide no such training. These conditions have improved since 1971 (see Chapter 11).

Only 15 percent of 102 respondents indicated that they have a major problem recruiting or retaining driver/attendants, and most attributed this to an insufficient number of available personnel in their area. Others cited the low pay scale for commercial services, the lack of individuals with a career interest in emergency care, the absence of suitable career ladders, and the lack of candidates meeting employment standards.

The majority of services do not utilize formal recruitment methods but rely instead on the initiative of current employees, word of mouth, and informal scouting. The most fruitful source of new driver/attendants is through other functions of the ambulance organization. Many services, especially municipal and volunteer fire or police departments, hire driver/attendants from the ranks of their own employees (or volunteers) assigned to other tasks.

The driver/attendant work force varies in duration of service. Of 128 respondent services, 86 percent indicated that on the average their personnel are employed for three years or more. Commercial services have a faster turnover, with approximately 20 percent employing personnel on the average of one year or less.

VEHICLES AND EQUIPMENT

There are 200 vehicles operated as emergency ambulances in Connecticut (excluding forty-two rescue trucks), and all are ground ambulances. In extreme cases, emergency service can be provided by Civil Air Patrol aircraft. Approximately two-thirds are custom ambulances (i.e., Cadillac, Oldsmobile, or Pontiac models). Twelve percent are hearses which are also used as ambulances. The rest are some type of van, converted station wagon, or converted panel truck. Utilization of rescue trucks was mentioned by ten emergency services (eight light rescue trucks and two heavy). Light rescue trucks are usually employed for extrication procedures but are used to transport emergency patients only if an ambulance is unavailable. (For a more complete discussion of this subject, see Chapter 4.)

Commercial services average 2.6 emergency vehicles each, of which approximately 75 percent are the custom variety. Volunteer and municipal services average 1.2 and 1.5 emergency vehicles each, respectively, and these are also predominantly custom ambulances. The municipal police departments operate eighteen of the nineteen converted station wagons, most of which service a dual function as patrol cars.

A significant percentage of emergency ambulances (19 percent) were manufactured in the year of the survey (1971), and an additional 41 percent were less than three years old. Approximately 40 percent were older than five years. (The U.S. Department of Transportation recommends that vehicles older than five years be replaced.) The majority of new vehicles are custom ambulances and station wagons, many of which are traded in every six or twelve months under leasing arrangements.

A number of variables could be considered in assessing the design of an effective emergency vehicle. Eleven U.S. Department of Transportation criteria were inventoried in this study (see Table 3-2). Seven of the eleven elements were present in 85 percent of vehicles, but 15 percent were not even clearly identified as ambulances (i.e., with the word "ambulance" and an emergency symbol such as a red cross). Only 62 percent of vehicles satisfied the patient compartment headroom criteria of 54 inches or higher. Municipal services were most deficient in this regard, especially the municipal police departments utilizing converted station wagons. Although most vehicles are heated, only 25 percent are air-conditioned.

The medical supplies and equipment carried on ambulances were inventoried (see Table 3-3). The majority of vehicles carry such basic first-aid items as gauze pads and dressings, triangular and roller bandages, adhesive tape, safety pins, and bandage shears. But portable suction, bag-mask ventilation units, and oropharyngeal airways are not carried on all vehicles—serious omissions, since these are essential to adequate emergency care. Additional essential supplies include disposable obstetrical kits (37 percent), poison kits (23 percent), and aluminum foil utilized for chest wounds (20 percent). The commercial services tend to carry more of these items, but none carries every item recommended by the Committee on Trauma of the American College of Surgeons.

Of the immobilizing equipment, inflatable splints are found on 85 percent of the vehicles and wood or metal splints on 7 percent. Only 40 percent of the vehicles carry hinged half-ring splints, and 56 percent carry long or short spine boards.

A stethoscope and blood-pressure cuff are carried on 55 percent of the commercial, 21 percent of the volunteer, and 14 percent of the

Table 3-2.   Emergency Vehicle Compliance with Minimal Standard Ambulance Design Criteria by Purveyor

| | Ambulance Purveyor | | | | | | | |
| Design Criteria | Commercial Vehicles[a] (n=74=100%) | | Volunteer Vehicles[b] (n=65=100%) | | Municipal Vehicles[c] (n=61=100%) | | Total Vehicles[d] (n=200=100%) | |
	Number	Percent	Number	Percent	Number	Percent	Number	Percent
Identified as an ambulance	63	85	59	91	47	77	169	85
Revolving (red) light	72	97	63	97	60	98	195	98
Flashing side/corner lights	72	97	60	92	52	85	194	97
Sealed underneath to prevent engine flooding	74	100	65	100	61	100	200	100
Four-wheel drive	0	—	1	2	0	—	1	0
Partitioned between patient and driver	72	97	61	94	39	64	172	86
Reinforced chassis in patient compartment	56	76	49	75	36	59	141	71
71" wide, 116" long, and 54" high inside patient compartment	52	70	43	66	29	48	124	62
Equipped with crash-stable fasteners to secure litters	71	96	62	95	59	97	192	96
Equipped with heater in patient area	74	100	63	97	52	85	189	95
Air-conditioned	30	41	12	19	8	3	50	25

[a]Under auspices of 28 commercial ambulance services (93%).
[b]Under auspices of 53 volunteer ambulance services (84%).
[c]Under auspices of 42 municipal ambulance services (88%).
[d]Under auspices of a total of 123 ambulance services (87%).

Source: Partial list recommended by Committee on Ambulance Design Criteria, National Academy of Engineering, in *Ambulance Design Criteria Manual* (Washington, D.C.: U.S. Department of Transportation, National Highway Safety Bureau, February 1970).

municipal vehicles. Many of the driver/attendants expressed a reluctance to use or even carry this equipment, indicating that their use should be limited to a physician or registered nurse. The technique of blood-pressure monitoring can readily be acquired by driver/attendants and would prove invaluable in helping to determine a patient's condition. With more advanced training of ambulance personnel, additional supplies, and equipment such as sterile intravenous agents, tracheal intubation kits, tracheostomy sets, venous cut-down sets, minor surgery kits, portable cardioscopes, defibrillators, and certain drugs might be utilized.

Table 3-3 reveals that many Connecticut ambulance services do not carry such essential items as oropharyngeal airways, portable suction apparatus, bag-mask ventilation units, and spine boards. Generally, municipal services are most lacking in this regard, but all services need to be upgraded with respect to basic equipment and supplies.

Few ambulances carry light rescue equipment. Although 63 percent of all vehicles carry pry bars, 74 percent carry jacks, and 51 percent carry tool kits, extrication equipment such as torches, wire cutters, and saws are included on less than one-fourth of the vehicles.

Equipment checklists, which were completed for 200 emergency vehicles, revealed that only five vehicles lacked two-way radios. But many of the radio-equipped vehicles provide for communication between the ambulance driver/attendant and his dispatcher only, and not directly with the hospital emergency department (see Chapter 4).

ORGANIZATION

The sixty-three volunteer and forty-eight municipal ambulance services that participated in the study are nonprofit organizations. Of the thirty commercial services, seven are individually owned, two are partnerships, and twenty-one are listed as corporations. Of the commercial firms, thirteen are solely involved in providing ambulance service, while seventeen have other business interests (see Table 3-4).

Approximately 20 percent of the ambulance services (volunteer and municipal) do no formal advertising. Of the 113 ambulance organizations that do advertise, 91 have a listing in the white and/or yellow pages of the telephone book. Of these, 22 advertise by business cards and fund drives and the remainder solely by word of mouth.

Connecticut ambulance organizations are affiliated with several professional ambulance associations. All the commercial firms belong

Table 3-3. Minimal Standard Medical and First-Aid Equipment Carried by Emergency Ambulances by Purveyor

| | Ambulance Purveyor | | | | | | | |
| | Commercial Vehicles[a] (n=74=100%) | | Volunteer Vehicles[b] (n=65=100%) | | Municipal Vehicles[c] (n=61=100%) | | Total Vehicles[d] (n=200=100%) | |
Minimal Standard Equipment	Number	Percent	Number	Percent	Number	Percent	Number	Percent
Portable oxygen unit	72	97	62	95	60	98	195	97
Portable suction apparatus	66	89	54	83	42	69	162	81
Bag-mask ventilation unit	66	89	45	69	42	69	153	77
Oropharyngeal airways	70	95	55	85	40	66	165	83
Mouth-to-mouth artificial ventilation airways	69	93	52	80	53	87	174	87
Mouth gags	65	88	32	49	25	41	122	61
Poison kit	16	22	20	31	10	16	46	23
Blood-pressure cuff with gauge	40	54	8	12	5	8	53	27
Stethoscope	42	57	20	31	13	21	75	38
Adhesive tape	66	89	62	95	57	93	185	93
Triangular bandages	66	89	62	95	53	87	181	91

Soft roller bandages	70	95	63	97	54	89	187	94
Sterile gauze pads (4" × 4")	70	95	63	97	56	92	189	95
Universal dressings	69	93	60	92	48	79	177	89
Bandage shears	70	95	59	91	47	77	176	88
Safety pins, large	66	89	54	83	46	75	166	83
Hinged half-ring splint	40	54	26	40	13	21	79	40
Wood or metal splints	57	77	41	63	36	59	134	67
Inflatable splints	57	77	60	92	52	85	169	85
Short spine board	47	64	37	57	25	41	109	55
Long spine board	57	77	36	55	24	39	117	59
Disposable obstetrical kit	41	55	21	32	12	20	74	37
Aluminum foil	25	34	6	9	8	13	39	20

[a] Under auspices of 28 commercial ambulance services (93%).
[b] Under auspices of 53 volunteer ambulance services (84%).
[c] Under auspices of 42 municipal ambulance services (88%).
[d] Under auspices of a total of 123 ambulance services (87%).

Source: Partial list approved by Committee on Trauma of the American College of Surgeons, May 1970.

Table 3-4.   Operation of Emergency Ambulance Service with Another Business by Commercial Ambulance Services

Other Business	Commercial Ambulance Services	
	Number	Percent
Funeral home	4	13
Hospital	1	3
Livery	2	7
Medical supply	2	7
Oxygen distributor	3	10
School bus	1	3
Service station	1	3
Taxi	3	10
None	13	43
Total	30	99

to the Connecticut Ambulance Association. Only sixteen of the forty-two volunteer services are members of the Connecticut Volunteer Ambulance Association, and several of them described their participation as "inactive." The fire department ambulance services are members of the Connecticut County Fire Chiefs Association. Several others are associated with loosely formed local emergency mutual-aid organizations that have been developed in an effort to pool emergency ambulance resources in rural areas. Two commercial services belong to the National Ambulance and Medical Service Association (NAMSA), and one commercial and two volunteer services are members of the International Rescue and First Aid Association. Thus only fifty-eight ambulance services, more than half of them commercial, participate in ambulance associations, and most of these described their participation as minimal.

Of 141 respondent ambulance organizations, 117 have some type of agreement with local municipalities, hospitals, and other ambulance services for the delivery of emergency medical care. Agreements with the municipalities involve contracts for the provision of emergency ambulance service to the residents of those particular towns. In addition, the municipalities impose standards of safety, sanitation, vehicle inspection, and quality of services on 20 ambulance services. Agreements with the hospitals involve admission policies for ambulance patients and/or transfer arrangements of patients to other emergency facilities. (Certain Hartford and New Haven hospitals have arrangements with local commercial purveyors who are called on a rotation basis.)

Almost half the present emergency ambulance services (including 60 percent of commercial firms and 56 percent of municipal services) have been in operation for more than twenty years. There is little variation among those purveyor groups in operation less than fifteen years: 37 percent are commercial, 40 percent volunteer, and 27 percent municipal. Of these, only one commercial and one municipal service have functioned for less than one year.

In the year prior to the study, twelve commercial purveyors stated that they had considered discontinuing their emergency ambulance service, compared to four volunteer and eight municipal services. The major reasons given were lack of qualified personnel, financial difficulties, and federal legislative standards such as the 1966 Fair Labor Standards Act.

OPERATIONAL POLICIES

As mentioned earlier, nearly all Connecticut emergency ambulance services will dispatch a vehicle for a traffic accident or any other type of emergency. The majority (89 percent) send two driver/attendants on all vehicles dispatched. But twelve services dispatch ambulances manned only by one driver/attendant. The reasons cited were insufficient standby personnel (eight services), lack of time to locate another trained driver/attendant (three services), and the requirement for a doctor's approval (one service). Only three of these twelve services (all municipal police departments) send one driver/attendant as a standard operating procedure. The need for two trained driver/attendants on each emergency ambulance run is obvious. Moreover, if a patient needs cardio-pulmonary resuscitation, then it is desirable to have at least three attendants (two in the patient compartment).

Because 65 percent of all Connecticut purveyors have only one ambulance, we inquired about their response to multiple requests for emergency assistance. In these circumstances, 56 percent of the purveyors transfer the call to a neighboring ambulance service, while 15 percent use standby equipment and personnel. If more than one request is received at a time, 17 percent will respond to the most urgent call first. Only 6 percent of the purveyors advise the caller to locate another service, 2 percent delay the second call until the first is completed, and 1 percent ($n = 2$) say that service is unavailable (2 percent are unknown).

Prompt and effective care must be given at the scene and en route to the hospital if a patient is to benefit maximally. In serious cases, approximately 93 percent of the services administer emergency care

Table 3-5.   First-Aid Techniques that Ambulance Driver/Attendants Are Trained to Perform, by Purveyor

	Ambulance Purveyor							
	Commercial (n=29)		Volunteer (n=60)		Municipal (n=46)		Total (n=135)	
First-Aid Technique	Number	Percent	Number	Percent	Number	Percent	Number	Percent
Administer oxygen	27	93	48	80	36	78	111	82
Care for burns	27	93	46	77	31	67	104	77
Control hemorrhaging	27	93	46	77	33	72	106	79
Control shock	26	90	46	77	31	67	103	76
Dress open wounds	27	93	47	78	34	74	108	80
Establish and maintain airways	26	90	45	75	31	67	102	76
Perform closed chest cardiac massage	26	90	44	73	30	65	100	74
Splint fractures	25	86	48	80	33	72	106	79

before the patient is transferred to the ambulance, and 89 percent provide care in the ambulance en route to the hospital. One-third of the services reported that initial care is often administered by someone else (usually police or fire department rescue units) before the ambulance arrives.

The ambulance purveyors were asked if their driver/attendants are trained to perform eight fundamental first-aid techniques (see Table 3-5). It is disturbing that none of the eight is performed by more than 82 percent of Connecticut ambulance personnel (including the establishing and maintaining of an airway, controlling hemorrhage, and administering oxygen). There has been significant improvement since 1971 as the result of EMT training.

The critical question of which hospital to transport an emergency patient depends on the following factors: time and distance to the nearest hospital; patient's condition; type of injury; patient's or family's request; preference of the ambulance driver/attendant, the assisting police or fire department rescue unit, or an attending physician; and agreement between the ambulance services and the hospitals. Most municipalities and ambulance purveyors have no set policy regarding hospital choice, and only 25 of the 141 purveyors feel there is a need for such a policy in their service area (see Chapters 4, 6, 10, and 11).

Approximately 76 percent of the purveyors inspect their medical equipment and first-aid supplies at least once a day, and 61 percent monitor equipment after each ambulance run. Some make inspections on a weekly or a monthly basis only, while others do so on a "regular" basis ranging anywhere from once a day to once a month.

A vehicle inspection is performed at least once a day by 61 percent of the purveyors, and 28 percent make checks after each run. Twenty-five percent of the volunteer and 21 percent of the municipal services conduct checks on a weekly basis.

Of the 141 respondent purveyors, only 55 percent keep a record of each ambulance run that includes the patient's name, address, destination, time of pickup, time of discharge, complaint, treatment rendered by ambulance crew, and source of the emergency call (see Table 3-6). While 95 percent of the services record patient's name, address, and destination, only 69 percent specify the chief complaint, and only 60 percent note the treatment rendered by the ambulance crew. Table 3-6 reveals that there is little variation between the major purveyor groups in recording most of these statistics. Another glaring deficiency in data recording is that 80 percent of the ambulance services interviewed do not even classify their runs by type of emergency.

Table 3–6.   Ambulance Records Kept by Purveyor

	Ambulance Purveyor							
	Commercial (n=30)		Volunteer (n=63)		Municipal (n=48)		Total (n=141)	
Statistics	*Number*	*Percent*	*Number*	*Percent*	*Number*	*Percent*	*Number*	*Percent*
Patient's name	29	97	45	94	60	95	134	95
Patient's address	29	97	45	94	60	95	134	95
Patient's destination	29	97	47	98	58	92	134	95
Time of pickup	25	83	40	83	54	86	119	84
Time of patient's discharge	25	83	40	83	54	86	119	84
Chief complaint	18	60	33	69	46	73	97	69
Treatment rendered by ambulance crew	12	40	28	58	44	70	84	60
Source of call	25	83	44	92	49	78	118	84
All the above statistics	14	47	23	48	40	67	77	55

PERFORMANCE TIMES

Figure 3–2 illustrates the components of emergency ambulance run time. (See Chapter 4 for a more detailed discussion of this subject.) A rough estimate of performance times is reflected by mean and median dispatch, response, and service times for immediate-dispatch and on-call vehicles. While these performance times are averages estimated by the individual purveyor, they closely approximate actual times as measured in the prospective study.

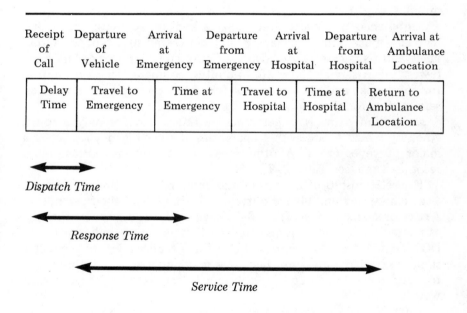

Figure 3-2. Performance Time for Ambulance Services

According to the data provided by purveyors, the mean elapsed time between when they receive the call for an ambulance and when the vehicle leaves the station (dispatch time) varies between 1.3 to 1.8 minutes for immediate-dispatch vehicles and between 5.3 and 8 minutes for on-call dispatch vehicles. The mean dispatch time for all immediate-dispatch vehicles is 1.4 minutes, compared to the DOT standard of 1 minute; the mean dispatch time for on-call vehicles is 5.4 minutes, compared to the DOT standard of 5 minutes.

The estimated mean elapsed time between receipt of a call and arrival of the ambulance at the scene of the emergency (response time) is 9.3 minutes for all purveyors. Commercial and municipal services have the lowest estimated response time—7.3 minutes for commercial and 8.3 minutes for municipal services, compared to 12.2 minutes for volunteers. The mean and median response times are well below the DOT standard, which stipulates a maximum of 30 minutes.

Ambulance purveyors were also asked to estimate mean and median service time—the elapsed time between dispatch of the ambulance and its release at the hospital. Commercial services estimate the lowest mean service time—26.3 minutes, compared to 32.5 minutes for municipal and 37.4 minutes for volunteer services. The mean service time for all purveyors is 33.1 minutes

Estimation of average performance times provides only a rough guide by which to assess the capabilities of an emergency service or a major purveyor group. Another measure is the estimated maximum response time (see Table 3-7).

The relationship of estimated maximum response time of Connecticut emergency ambulance purveyors to the size of their emergency service area is shown in Table 3-7. In general, the data show that the estimated maximum response time in Connecticut is in line with the DOT standard of 30 minutes. While three services do not meet this standard, in large measure their long maximum response time is due to poor access roads and long distances traveled (15-20 miles each way).

Further analysis reveals that the estimated maximum response time is inversely proportional to the population density of an individual town—i.e., the greater the population density, the lower the maximum response time. Causative factors affecting response time include distance to the emergency, road conditions, location of ambulance facilities, and dispatch capabilities of the emergency service.

DOT EVALUATION CRITERIA
AND SUMMARY OF FINDINGS

Although not totally complete, the criteria developed by the U.S. Department of Transportation (DOT) are useful in evaluating basic elements of emergency ambulance service. For the most part, these criteria are *minimum* standards and do not reflect the optimum.

Based on the DOT criteria listed in Table 3-8, chi-square testing indicated that there are no significant differences ($p < 0.100$) between commercial, volunteer, and municipal services in Connecticut. Overall compliance by Connecticut emergency ambulance services is clearly below par. For instance, only 22 percent of all services require an advanced Red Cross certificate before they will hire a driver/attendant. Performance is also poor in terms of emergency vehicles and equipment. Only three purveyors carry the six "essential" rescue items recommended by the American College of Surgeons on all emergency vehicles, and none of the services carries both the essential first-aid supplies and medical equipment *and* the rescue equipment items. The clear need for improvement in emergency ambulance services in Connecticut is highlighted by the fact that not one such service meets all the criteria approved by the National Highway Traffic Safety Administration of the U.S. Department of Transportation.

Table 3-7. Size of Emergency Service Area vs. Estimated Maximum Response Time for All Purveyors (n=141=100%)

Size of Emergency Service Area (Sq. Mi.)	Estimated Maximum Response Time (min.)															
	5		5-9		10-14		15-19		20-24		25-29		30 or more		Total	
	Num-ber	Per-cent	Num-ber	Per-cent	Num-ber	Per-cent	Num-ber	Per-cent	Num-ber	Per-cent	Num-ber	Per-cent	Num-ber	Per-cent	Num-ber	Per-cent
10			9	50	4	6									13	9
10-24			9	50	29	45	3	12	1	4					42	30
25-49					27	42	13	72	3	12					43	30
50-74					2	3	2	8	1	4					5	4
75-99					1	2	6	24	6	24					13	9
100-49					1	2	1	4	10	40					12	9
150-99									4	16					4	3
200-49											5	83	2	67	7	5
250-99											1	17			1	1
300-99															—	—

400–99													1	33	1	1
500 or more	—	18	100	64	100	25	100	25	100	6	100	3	100	1	141	101
Total	—	18	100	64	100	25	100	25	100	6	100	3	100	1	33	1

Note: Estimated Maximum Response Time is the estimated time between receipt of an emergency call and arrival of the ambulance at the farthest point (from the specific ambulance purveyor station) in the emergency service area.

Assumptions:

1. Linear travel at 25 miles per hour in areas of population density greater than 500 people per square mile.[a]
2. Linear travel at 40 miles per hour in areas of population density less than 500 people per square mile.[b]
3. Dispatch time for immediate-dispatch vehicles is 1 minute.[c]
4. Dispatch time of on-call dispatch vehicles is 5 minutes.[c]

Sources:

[a] Paul Joseph Brown, "Fire Department Medical Emergency Van Evaluation and System Simulation," master's thesis, Yale University, New Haven, Connecticut, 1970, p. 69. This study concluded that average linear speed for an emergency ambulance in areas of population density greater than 500 people per square mile is 25 miles per hour.

[b] Dunlap and Associates, Inc., *New Hampshire Ambulance Services: Current Status and Planning Requirements* (1970), p. 60. This study concluded that average linear speed for an emergency ambulance in New Hampshire is 40 miles per hour. Since most of New Hampshire has a population density of less than 500 people per square mile, we decided to utilize the 40 mile per hour figure to measure linear speed in sections of Connecticut where population density is less than 500 people per square mile.

[c] Maximum dispatch times recommended by the U.S. Department of Transportation.

Table 3–8.   Connecticut Emergency Ambulance Services Meeting the National Highway Traffic Safety Administration Funding Criteria, by Purveyor

Funding Criteria	Ambulance Purveyor							
	Commercial		Volunteer		Municipal		Total	
	Number	Percent	Number	Percent	Number	Percent	Number	Percent
Two driver/attendants on all emergency runs (n=137=97%)	29	97	57	92	39	85	125	88
24-hour coverage by emergency ambulance and personnel (n=141=100%)	30	100	63	100	48	100	141	100
One minute or less dispatch for immediate-dispatch vehicles; 5 minutes or less for on-call vehicles (n=105=75%)	17	68	32	73	24	67	73	70
Advanced Red Cross Certificate required of new driver/attendants before hiring (n=132=94%)	27	90	63	100	48	100	138	98
All emergency vehicles meet selected design criteria (except four-wheel drive) (n=123=87%)	8	29	14	23	7	16	29	22
All emergency vehicles equipped with "essential" medical equipment items (n=123=87%)	5	18	8	15	2	5	15	12
All emergency vehicles equipped with essential rescue-equipment items (n=123=87%)	1	4	1	2	—	—	2	2
All emergency vehicles equipped with two-way radio (n=141=100%)	—	—	2	4	1	2	3	2
Fulfill all above criteria (n=105=75%)	29	97	59	94	48	100	136	97

�֍ *Appendix 3A*

Estimating Ambulance Call Volume

A regression model was employed to estimate total ambulance and emergency call volumes on the basis of area population:

Annual Number of Ambulance Calls

Population of Town	*Emergencies*	*Total Calls*
≤ 30,000	$y = 14.54x + 43.52$	$y = 22.23x + 52.98$
> 30,000	$y = 31.82x - 569.29$	$y = 47.98x - 725.02$

where x = population (in thousands)
y = number of calls.

These equations were utilized to estimate the emergency and total ambulance call volumes expected for Connecticut communities. On the basis of 1970 census data and the prospective and retrospective ambulance surveys, Connecticut's 1970 ambulance call volume is estimated to be 101,535, including 65,770 calls that would be classified by purveyors as emergency calls. This volume is equivalent to one ambulance call per day per 10,925 population.

There are two other readily available sources of ambulance call volume. One is the popular rule-of-thumb measure often used by commercial services of one ambulance call per day per 10,000 population. The other source is the call data compiled through a special study by the Connecticut Department of Health in fiscal year 1970, which produced an estimate of one call per day per 9,041 people. However, if data from this source are given by type of call and if the entire column by type of call is summed (no estimate of dry runs given), the total number of calls for Connecticut is 99,257, or one call per day per 11,176 population. These alternative sources are admittedly difficult to compare, but our study volumes are conservative estimates of ambulance service demand. They can be regarded as the minimal number of calls per year that should be expected by ambulance purveyors.

Table 3A–1 compares ambulance call volumes estimated from the alternative sources discussed above.

Table 3A-1. Estimates of 1970 Calls in Connecticut—Comparison of Sources

	EAS Calls		
	Emergency	Total	1 Call/Day/ Population
1971 Study Regression Model	65,770	101,535	10,925
Connecticut Department of Health	70,408	99,257[a]	11,176
Connecticut Department of Health	70,408	122,702	9,041
Rule-of-Thumb Measure	—	110,932	10,000

[a]Based on the actual sum of each type of call reported (dry runs excluded).

✳ *Chapter 4*

Emergency Medical Communications

INTRODUCTION AND OBJECTIVES

The full benefits of improved emergency medical services will not be realized if the citizen has difficulty in gaining access to them because of poor communications systems. In addition to ambulance services and hospital emergency departments, other services such as police, fire, and civil defense frequently have important roles in EMS and all should be able to communicate directly with each other in order to assure prompt, high quality emergency care. Good emergency medical communications serve as the glue that holds the other elements of the EMS system together.

This chapter begins with an analysis of the concepts of "critical time," "entry time," and "response time." The typical patterns of communication between Connecticut citizens and various emergency agencies are summarized and data are presented concerning: citizen entry into the system, coordination of communications capability between emergency services, and clinical communication between physicians and ambulance personnel at the emergency scene. A regression formula to estimate the volume of emergency medical calls is then presented. The chapter concludes with a proposed regional emergency medical response system—one that is tailored to the south central region of Connecticut but could serve as a model for any region.

THE CONCEPT OF "CRITICAL TIME"

From the perspective of the patient, any time that is lost before emergency care is rendered at the emergency scene may be critical to the patient's chances of recovery. This "critical time" is the period between the time a person first seeks emergency medical help and the arrival of the appropriate emergency vehicle and personnel at the scene, where initial aid can be given.

Critical time has two major components—"entry time" and "response time" (see Figure 4-1). Entry time begins when emergency medical assistance is first sought and continues until someone is contacted who has the authority and ability to take direct action by dispatching an ambulance with trained personnel. This includes the time taken in ascertaining location, determining what emergency service to call, placing the call (which often involves one or more transfers or redialing), and making voice contact with the appropriate person or agency.

The second component—response time—begins only when the person with the authority to dispatch an ambulance receives the call and ends when appropriate qualified assistance arrives on the emergency scene. This includes interpreting the call, selecting the appropriate response vehicle, dispatching the vehicle (and giving medical advice to the caller where feasible and appropriate), as well as the vehicle's

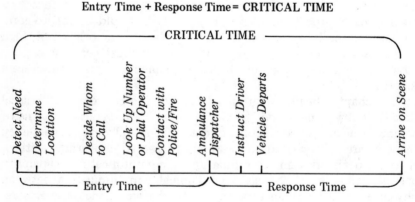

Figure 4-1. Critical Time in Emergency Medical Services

travel time to the emergency scene.

Most of the literature and analysis regarding this area (particularly the discussion in public arenas) is limited to response time, in part because it is more easily measurable. Indeed, hard data accurately measuring entry time are probably impossible to obtain. The difficulty of measurement notwithstanding, an ideal system of emergency medical communications should contain no elements that unnecessarily lengthen either entry time or response time and should contain no unnecessary relaying of vital medical information that might increase the likelihood of error.

AN OVERVIEW OF EMERGENCY MEDICAL COMMUNICATIONS IN CONNECTICUT

There is no doubt that the technology exists to build a strong EMS communications system, but in most of Connecticut, as in most of the nation, such well-planned systems simply did not exist when we undertook our study.[a] In Connecticut, there are a variety of sources that the public can call for assistance, although they are often not readily identified in telephone books or on pay telephones. In a few communities, the citizen can dial the 911 emergency telephone number, but in most areas this number is limited to police and fire services. Thus, the citizen frequently dials the operator, and a confusing and time-consuming process can begin that significantly lengthens entry time.

The following are examples of hazards that citizens may face in obtaining emergency care. After they recognize the need for urgent medical assistance, they may be unable to determine whom to call because no number is provided in the front of the telephone book or on the telephone itself. If they are at a pay phone without the change necessary to get a dial tone, additional delay results. If they dial the operator, they may reach someone located far away who is unfamiliar with their location. If they are strangers to the region or are in a rural area, they may not be able to identify their location because this information is not usually provided on the telephone instrument.

---

[a]Impediments to implementation have been primarily administrative, jurisdictional, and economic, and, as seen in Chapter 1, the recent national efforts to build regional systems are beginning to address these problems. For additional analysis of implementation problems, see: American Hospital Association, "A Guide for Hospital Participation in an Emergency Medical Communications System," Chicago, Illinois, 1973.

Once these barriers are crossed, the operator may transfer the call to the local police department. In some cases, the police are unable to handle the call and transfer it again; in others, the police dispatcher may dispatch a patrol car to verify that an ambulance is necessary. In the latter case, the patrolman arrives at the scene, determines that a true emergency exists, and then calls the dispatcher to request an ambulance. The police dispatcher then calls an ambulance dispatcher, in many cases without knowing whether the ambulance service is already occupied on other emergency calls and thus not immediately available.

Finally, the ambulance is dispatched to "respond" to the request, and here "response time" begins. If, at the scene, the ambulance attendant needs medical advice or wishes to notify the emergency facility of the patient's condition prior to arrival, the attendant must inform the dispatcher by radio, and the dispatcher in turn must contact the hospital emergency department (often by telephone) to relay the messages.

There are many variations to this flow, but our study data indicate that the aforementioned patterns are frequent. Additional uncertainties confront the citizen when a fire department or civil defense is involved; when several uncoordinated ambulance services exist in an area; or when there is no policy about the disposition of special emergencies such as burns, spinal-cord injuries, or head-trauma cases.[b]

Following this background, we now turn to a review of emergency medical communications in Connecticut.

DATA ANALYSIS

To obtain information about communications regarding Connecticut EMS, we employed two data-collection techniques. One was an interview survey document developed for hospitals and ambulance services. The other was a mailed questionnaire for police and fire departments designed to obtain information about emergency-call reception and response activities (see Chapter 2).

---

[b]For example, if a citizen calls either the Hospital of St. Raphael or Yale-New Haven Hospital in New Haven and requests an ambulance, he will be referred to one of several private ambulance companies *on a rotation basis* and without regard to whether it is the closest or most appropriate vehicle. This policy has been mandated by the ambulance companies who are concerned about "losing" any calls.

Data gathered from ambulance, police, fire, and hospital services address three components: citizen entry (the process by which a person enters the system), communications operations (the coordination between all emergency services), and clinical consultation (involving two-way radio/voice communications between ambulance personnel at the scene or en route to the hospital and the emergency department).

Citizen Entry

Police and fire agencies receive most of their requests for emergency medical assistance via telephone directly from a citizen (see Table 4-1). In contrast, ambulance companies receive only 21 percent of their calls from a citizen; most calls are relayed via telephone from police, fire, community telephone operators, physicians, and hospitals.

Of the 140 ambulance services responding, 45 have no listed telephone number in local telephone directories. Only 58 list their services in the front of local directories along with other emergency numbers, while the remaining 37 list their services only in the yellow or white pages. Because all police and fire departments have easily identifiable emergency listings, citizens under stress often elect to call these services or the telephone operator rather than ambulance companies.

Thirty-two ambulance services require confirmation by a policeman, fireman, or physician before responding to a citizen's request for assistance in order to assure that an emergency ambulance is necessary. The benefits of eliminating the use of an emergency vehicle for routine transport must be weighed against the ensuing delay in arrival of qualified medical assistance at the scene when a true emergency exists.

Coordination of Communications Services

Upon receipt of a request for emergency assistance, an agency's response is often dependent on its links with other agencies as well as its own capabilities. Nearly half of the police and fire agencies do not respond directly to an emergency request but relay the information to another agency (see Table 4-2).

To understand the working relationships among police, fire, and ambulance services, it is important to distinguish between rescue and ambulance operations. Some overlap of functions between these services has always existed and will undoubtedly continue. Although all fire services perceive their primary mission as fire fighting, all recognize some role in extricating injured or burned people from the

Table 4–1. Source of Emergency Call Compared with Type of EMS Agency (by percentage)

Caller	State Police (n=51=100%)	Local Police (n=72=100%)	Fire Departments (n=168=100%)	Ambulances (n=140=100%)	Hospitals (n=37=100%)
Citizen[a]	82	61	47	21	8
Police	10	19	14	28	32
Fire	—	—	10	12	11
Ambulance	—	—	—	—	22
Hospital[b]	—	6	1	4	—
Community telephone operator	—	—	6	11	—
Answering service	2	—	1	4	—
Physician	—	8	5	11	—
Not notified	—	—	—	—	16
No pattern	6	6	16	9	11

[a] Anyone other than policemen, firemen, telephone operators, hospital staff, or physicians.
[b] Includes two Veterans Administration hospitals.

Table 4-2. Comparison of Direct Dispatch and Information Relay, by Agency

Agency	Dispatches Assistance Directly		Relays Information to Another Agency	
	Number	Percent	Number	Percent
State police (n=55)	24	44	31	56
Local police (n=72)	37	51	35	49
Fire departments (n=168)	88	52	80	48
Total	149	51	146	49

scene. Many fire services provide basic emergency medical measures such as resuscitation and splinting before turning the patient over to ambulance personnel for more advanced medical care and transport to the hospital. Some fire services include patient transportation and thus function as an ambulance service as well as a rescue service.

Because there are no generally accepted definitions of "ambulance" and "rescue" services, much of the data depend on the perception of the fire and police services themselves. For our purposes, a working definition of *rescue* services includes those that extricate a person from danger and provide basic emergency care when necessary at the scene but do *not* routinely transport the patient. (See Chapter 3, p. 63.)

Our data show that 55 percent of state police, 72 percent of local police, and 54 percent of fire departments dispatch rescue units through direct communication with vehicle drivers; while 25 percent, 15 percent, and 14 percent, respectively, relay this information. Table 4-3 compares the three types of services that are routinely provided when rescue units are dispatched directly. The most common procedure is to provide basic emergency medical assistance but not transportation. Table 4-3 also shows that many services, particularly fire services, operate ambulances as well. Although, in some cases the same vehicle serves both the rescue and ambulance function, in others, different vehicles are used.

Police and fire departments are much less involved in the direct dispatch of ambulance services than in initial rescue response. As Table 4-4 shows, the ambulance-dispatching capabilities of police and fire agencies are often limited to a relay procedure either on receipt of the initial call or after the need is determined at the scene of the emergency.

Fire and local police departments have a greater capability than state police units in direct dispatching of ambulance services. The inability of many police and fire agencies to directly dispatch ambu-

Table 4–3. Comparison of Rescue Services Routinely Provided by Police and Fire Agencies

	State Police		Local Police		Fire Departments	
	Number	*Percent*	*Number*	*Percent*	*Number*	*Percent*
Provides neither emergency medical care nor transport of patients (assumed to be extrication only)[a]	4	14	14	30	12	13
Provides emergency medical care but not transport of patients[b]	15	57	24	52	57	63
Provides emergency medical care and transport of patients[c]	9	29	8	18	21	23
Total	28	100	46	100	90	99

[a]14 percent of these local police and 17 percent of these fire agencies reported operating ambulance services.

[b]12 percent of these local police and 16 percent of these fire agencies reported operating ambulance services.

[c]38 percent of these local police and 86 percent of these fire agencies reported operating ambulance services.

lance services is largely related to the wide variety of ambulance services (including commercial, volunteer, municipal, and hospital units) as well as police and fire departments (see Chapter 3). This diversity of control, authority, and jurisdiction has been a primary barrier to the integration of emergency medical communications into comprehensive systems. However, the dispatching role of police and

Table 4–4. Methods by Which Police and Fire Agencies Mobilize Ambulance Services (by percentage)

	State Police (n=51)	Local Police (n=72)	Fire Departments (n=164)
Direct dispatch	8	43	45
Relay information	53	42	23
From patrol car at scene	37	13	8
From rescue unit at scene	—	1	18
No ambulance—rescue vehicle used	—	—	1
No ambulance—patrol car used	2	1	1
Not indicated	—	—	4

fire departments should not be minimized—81 percent of municipal and 60 percent of volunteer ambulance services, indicate that police and fire agencies were responsible for their dispatching. In contrast, 90 percent of the commercial services have their own dispatchers, thereby inserting another individual into the relay pattern (the citizen's call is rarely made directly to the commercial service).

The actual locating and dispatching of ambulance drivers and attendants is an additional element in providing timely and efficient ambulance response. For almost half of the volunteer services, the drivers and attendants are not with the vehicle and they must be notified and assembled before the vehicle can respond. This notification is usually by telephone and may require several calls before an ambulance crew is assembled. Table 4-5 shows the variety of dispatch methods used by ambulance services, ranging from telephone and radio to in-person notification (instructions given to the driver directly by dispatcher who is at the same location).

To utilize resources optimally, it is important for ambulance services to integrate their services with police and fire departments. Although nearly all ambulance services have two-way radio equipment, their ability to contact other agencies directly varies considerably. Only 3 percent of volunteer and commercial and 10 percent of municipal ambulance services can contact all three relevant agencies in their service area—police, fire, and hospital—directly by radio.

Table 4-6 reveals that 76 percent of commercial ambulance companies have radio contact only with their own vehicles, whereas only 3 percent of volunteer and municipal services are so limited. Volunteer and municipal services have greater radio communications capability with other emergency service agencies than commercial providers.

Although 93 of the 169 towns surveyed have central dispatching of two or more emergency services, 81 of these are limited to single

Table 4-5. Driver Dispatching Methods Used, by Types of Ambulance Services (by percentage)

Procedure Used	Commercial (n=30)	Volunteer (n=76)	Municipal (n=33)	Hospital (n=1)
In-person	48	14	19	—
Radio	19	14	31	100
Telephone	10	46	28	—
Telephone/in-person/ radio (combination of 2)	16	12	19	—
Other	7	14	3	—

Table 4-6.   Comparison of Radio Communications Capability with Type of Ambulance Organization (by percentage)

Radio Links	Type of Organization			
	Commercial (n=29=100%)	Municipal (n=32=100%)	Volunteer (n=75=100%)	Hospital (n=1=100%)
Ambulance only	76	3	3	—
Ambulance/police	7	23	8	—
Ambulance/fire	—	23	40	—
Ambulance/fire/ police	7	32	36	—
Ambulance/hos- pital/police	—	6	3	100
Ambulance/hos- pital	7	3	4	—
Ambulance/hos- pital/fire/ police	3	10	3	—
Fire	—	—	1	—
Other	—	—	2	—

town areas. Of the remaining 12 central dispatch networks, 2 cover only 2 towns each, and 6 cover 3 towns each. In short, there is no health services area in Connecticut that has a truly integrated emergency medical service on a regionwide basis providing a single access point for citizen entry.

Clinical Consultation

In addition to communications needs discussed above, there is a need for clinical consultation to permit the transmission of medical advice and information between the emergency department and the emergency scene. This includes instances when the ambulance attendant advises the emergency department of the condition and impending arrival of a patient or requests a physician's advice regarding treatment of a patient at the scene or en route to the hospital. The latter case may require lengthy or frequent conversations between the attendant and the physician over two-way radio—unlike messages in the initial dispatch function, which are usually very short.

In-transit communications are useful to mobilize and prepare hospital support services during the transport of the emergency patient to the hospital emergency facility. Fifty-nine percent of the ambulance dispatchers "almost always" notify the hospital prior to arrival, and 34 percent give the hospital advance notification when transporting "serious cases." The remaining ambulance services (6 percent) seldom notify the hospital in advance or do so only upon request of the physician.

Most ambulance services (84 percent) contact hospitals via telephone, which can be a slow method because of relays through switchboard operators. As Table 4-7 shows, only 12 percent of the ambulance services have direct radio contact between their vehicles and hospital emergency departments. Whether a radio or telephone is used, 95 percent of the ambulance services believe the hospital's response to their arrival is enhanced with advance notification. Certainly, direct connection between principals is more desirable than relays through switchboards. Direct radio communication between ambulances and hospital emergency departments is necessary if attendants are to provide advanced levels of care based on physician supervision and advice.

Of the thirty-seven hospitals reporting, twenty-seven have some type of two-way radio equipment, and twenty-two of these use this equipment solely for "emergency medical services" or some combination of "emergency medical service," civil defense, and internal hospital communication needs. However, a large portion of the hospitals indicated that radio utilization for "emergency medical services" is limited to hospital-to-hospital communication; only 30 percent have radio communication with ambulance services. No hospital reported radio communication capability with all four essential agencies—police, fire, ambulance, and other hospitals.

Lack of two-way radio communication between hospitals and other agencies may be mitigated at the eighteen hospitals with hot lines (direct telephone lines that require no dialing and provide immediate contact) to both police and ambulance agencies. Although this technique eliminates delay in establishing two-party connections, it still requires a relay of information that would be eliminated if direct radio contact were available between the ambulance driver and emergency-department personnel.

Table 4-7. Procedure Utilized by Ambulance Services to Notify Hospital of Patient Arrival

Notification Procedure	Number of Services	Percentage of Services
Telephone hospital prior to pick-up	11	8
Radio from ambulance to hospital emergency department	17	12
Radio from ambulance to dispatcher, who telephones hospital	105	76
Radio from ambulance to dispatcher, who radios hospital	2	1
Other	4	3
Total	139	100

ESTIMATING THE VOLUME AND TYPE
OF EMERGENCY CALLS

To plan a comprehensive system of emergency medical response, it is essential to know the volume and type of calls received so that communication loads can be forecast. But many police and fire departments, like ambulance services, do not keep accurate records of the number and type of calls received. However, we do know that local police departments receive considerably more requests for all types of emergency assistance and for emergency medical assistance than state police and fire agencies. This higher call load relates directly to the larger populations served by local police departments. Many small Connecticut towns rely on resident state troopers and volunteer fire departments for their emergency services.

The volume of general emergency calls (police, fire, and medical) generated by a community is reasonably predictable. Based on data obtained from a separate study we made of thirty-one Connecticut towns, about 30 percent of all emergency calls are requests for medical assistance. The majority of the remainder are assumed to be for police assistance rather than fire, although no attempt was made to quantify this.

Recognizing that the great majority of emergency medical assistance calls go through police or fire departments, a regression formula was developed using police and fire data in ten towns with populations over 10,000.[c] Complete data were obtained for all thirty-one towns studied, but in the lower population groups there was poor correlation between the formula and actual data. Applying the formula to the ten towns and averaging the results, we found that one general emergency call (police, fire, or medical) per day occurs for every 3,400 people and that one emergency medical call per day occurs for every 11,000 people. Although this is not a sensitive measure of volume and does not take into account peak periods, it does provide a starting point for communities and regions to plan the type of emergency response resources they will need. These data correlate well with the call projections discussed in Appendix 3A.

A PROPOSED REGIONAL EMERGENCY
MEDICAL RESPONSE SYSTEM—
THE SOUTH CENTRAL
CONNECTICUT EXPERIENCE

The advantages of a regional response system with central dispatching and coordination of emergency medical resources become clear

[c]Call data on all thirty-one towns are included in Appendix 4A.

when compared with the uncoordinated communications just described. The advantages include:

1. Citizen access is improved and critical time (particularly entry time) reduced by providing a single, easily identified access number.
2. Ambulance services can be better utilized because resources in a region can be better allocated through central dispatching.
3. All emergency services—whether police, fire, or ambulance of any type—can be dispatched with equal efficiency and speed.
4. Because the emergency service area of hospital EDs covers an area served by several ambulance agencies, and because hospitals have varying levels of emergency service capability, the optimal routing of patients is best coordinated centrally (particularly if an acceptable categorization strategy for the region exists).
5. The central medical emergency dispatcher (CMED) could become a true medical professional, trained in triaging emergency problems over the telephone and knowledgeable enough to give initial medical advice where appropriate.
6. The removal of the need to relay information through several communication points reduces the likelihood of error and thus should improve the quality of care.
7. The cost of operating a regional response system can be spread over the entire region, and duplicative, unnecessary dispatch capabilities can be eliminated.

For these reasons and because regional systems had been successfully implemented in several other areas of the country, we constructed a plan for a regional system for the fifteen-town area in the south central part of the state. The region was chosen because of its proximity to the research team and because it contained the communications and medical characteristics typical of much of the state. The region includes two New Haven hospitals (Yale-New Haven and the Hospital of St. Raphael), a Veterans Administration hospital, a variety of ambulance services (commercial, municipal, and volunteer), and an uncoordinated potpourri of telephone numbers for requesting emergency medical assistance.

In New Haven, for example, emergency medical calls to the telephone operator or police end up at the fire department emergency switchboard, which dispatches a fire department rescue unit. This unit provides first aid at the scene and then makes a judgment regarding the need for further medical help by radioing a request back to the emergency switchboard dispatcher, who in turn contacts a private ambulance company dispatcher, who then dispatches an ambulance.

If a policemen arrives at the emergency scene first, he radios the police dispatcher to request an ambulance. The police dispatcher advises the emergency switchboard operator, who in turn contacts an ambulance service by tie-line telephone. The choice of ambulance service is made according to a rotation system rather than availability of the nearest ambulance.

Generally, the emergency system in the surrounding towns functions in the same manner as that in New Haven. With one exception (Guilford police), the emergency switchboard operators and police dispatchers have no direct communications with individual ambulances but must relay emergency messages through the ambulance dispatcher. To eliminate this fragmentation, duplication, and delay, we recommended that a CMED be established to coordinate all emergency medical services throughout the south central area of Connecticut served by the Yale-New Haven and St. Raphael Hospitals. The CMED and the related communications system would dispatch all emergency ambulances and rescue vehicles in the area and coordinate patient loads in hospital emergency departments.[1]

Through the use of a well-identified emergency medical number, entry time could be significantly reduced by the elimination of uncertainty about whom to call and transfers of calls. The CMED would also reduce response time by dispatching the closest and most appropriate ambulance to the scene. The CMED's impact on critical time is shown in Figure 4-2.

The CMED could be financed in part by proportional assessments based on the population of the participating communities and in part by a charge for each ambulance run. The operational cost of running a comprehensive ambulance service is very low, significantly lower than for police and fire services (see Chapter 5). Furthermore, some economies might result from the fact that each ambulance service would no longer need to maintain twenty-four-hour dispatch capability.[d] Initial capital costs for such items as base stations and mobile radios might be absorbed by federal or private foundation funds, but continuing operational costs should be borne by the region.

[d]Chapter 5 analyzes the many subsidies now in use to support ambulance services in Connecticut and makes a strong case for their expansion. Dispatching is one of the monetary-equivalent subsidies that municipalities provide for ambulance services. Of the monetary-equivalent subsidies received by sixty-seven purveyors, 15 percent were in the form of dispatching services. Many other municipalities could provide this service without a significant increase in cost, particularly if linked to an existing dispatch center such as the fire department.

Entry Time + Response Time = CRITICAL TIME

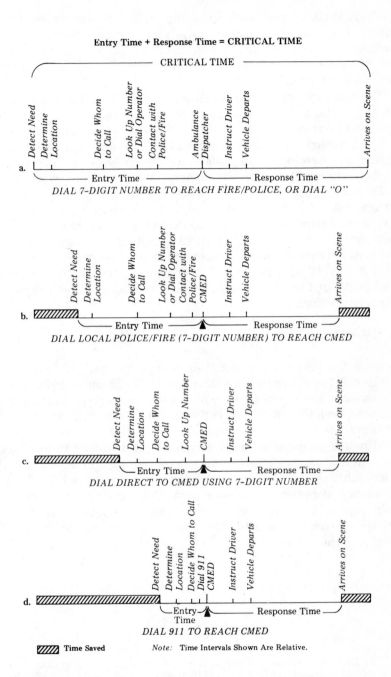

Figure 4-2. Methods of Obtaining Emergency Medical Assistance

The CMED concept was generally well received by physicians, police, fire, ambulance, and hospital personnel. Some volunteer ambulance services expressed concern about possible loss of identity and private companies expressed reservations about loss of control over their business.

The primary barriers to acceptance were the initial capital costs, the political questions of ultimate authority and control, and determination of responsibility for the long-term management of the system. All agreed that the concept was feasible and that, if the initial capital and developments costs could be covered, the prospects of implementation through a two-hospital consortium were good.[e]

To make maximum use of existing resources, other Connecticut regions will have to determine the most appropriate structure, location, and organization of a CMED. These decisions will be based on such factors as volume of emergency calls; links with police, fire, and civil defense services; number and type of hospitals; existence of UHF and VHF systems; population density; the size of the region; availability of the 911 emergency number; and political and jurisdictional considerations.

SUMMARY OF FINDINGS

In most Connecticut communities, there is no well-publicized number to call for emergency medical assistance. In many instances, the citizen calls the operator or police and fire agencies who are often not equipped to respond directly but must transfer the call to another agency.

Although most ambulance services have two-way radios linking their dispatcher and vehicles, only 5 percent of Connecticut's ambulance vehicles can communicate directly by radio with a hospital emergency department. No region in Connecticut has developed a truly integrated emergency medical response system that provides prompt citizen access and coordination of all emergency care resources in the region.

---

[e]Funding for developing a regional emergency medical communications system was obtained in 1974 from the Robert Wood Johnson Foundation (see Chapters 1 and 11).

Appendix 4A

Sample of Communities in Connecticut by Population Showing the Volume of Emergency Calls Received by Police and Fire Departments

Town Population	Total Emergency Calls Received in 1970 by Police and Fire Depts.	Portion of Total Calls Requesting Emergency Medical Assistance	
		Number	%
433	14	1	7%
1,022	26	8	30%
1,452	12	2	17%
1,609	5	1	20%
2,066	29	9	31%
2,673	47	16	35%
3,129	330	103	31%
3,593	50	20	40%
3,691	425	30	9%
3,748	98	28	27%
3,755	204	96	46%
3,815	55	15	27%
4,070	88	42	47%
4,911	60	15	25%
5,542	1119	732	65%
6,150	92	30	34%
6,895	200	30	15%
7,673	300	200	67%
7,857	450	215	48%
8,140	185	79	42%
8,468	1137	352	31%
10,267	688	446	65%
15,553	650	133	20%
18,188	2126	1183	55%
20,444	302	267	83%
27,414	7256	1837	26%
36,523	8703	2470	29%
49,357	13083	1029	8%
57,583	2152	862	33%
137,707	11452	4710	41%
156,542	9838	4149	42%

Totals:

622,280	60,825	19,119	31%

※ *Chapter 5*

Costs of Emergency
Ambulance Services

INTRODUCTION AND OBJECTIVES

As health planners and decisionmakers across the country consider how best to provide emergency medical services, they must address the question: at what cost? Unfortunately, there are very little useful data on the costs of ambulance services or on the cost of care in the hospital emergency department (ED). We found it particularly difficult to obtain cost data in Connecticut. Indeed, our efforts concerning ED costs were so unproductive that we could draw no substantive conclusions concerning them.

In our attempt to investigate ED costs, we collected statements of direct and indirect costs from all hospitals in the state. This included an analysis of physician, nursing, and other health professional salaries as well as a comparison of estimated total costs and total revenues over a ten-year period. A comparison of these costs and revenues was made according to type of physician reimbursement. Unfortunately, the necessity of using an accounting mechanism designed to measure inpatient costs biased the data generated and made them almost useless despite full cooperation from the hospitals. For example, we found that the method of allocating indirect costs was inappropriate and skewed the data so that there was no relationship between staffing mix, services provided, and cost.[1]

Although obtaining ambulance cost data was also difficult, through the methods to be discussed below, we were able to draw some conclusions. Some ambulance services kept no data at all while others maintained records in a manner that made comparisons difficult or impossible. Costing methodologies differed among providers and often were unacceptable. Even basic cost estimates were often lacking. Cooperation from providers was difficult and often impossible to obtain because of the fear that such information would be used against them by competitors or by regulatory agencies.[2]

Because of these obstacles, we focused our efforts on a fourteen-town area of the state where data were the most reliable and provider cooperation was particularly good. While the findings reported here are based on only a 28 percent sample of all purveyors (n=46), we believe the region reflects many of the important characteristics of ambulance services in Connecticut and the data provide useful insights into the nature and magnitude of their costs. This region contains fifteen commercial, sixteen municipal, and fifteen volunteer ambulance purveyors.

METHODOLOGY

We calculated the cost per run for each purveyor by dividing the total cost of operations for each by the number of trips made. A comparison of purveyors by class was made by calculating the percentage of fixed and variable expenses for each purveyor.

Costs per capita provided by different types and mixes of purveyors were calculated for all towns or cities in the study area. Total costs of operations for all purveyors in each municipality or service area plus profits for commercial operations and other tax-borne expenditures for municipal and volunteer services were totaled and divided by the population served. A comparison of costs per capita based upon type of purveyor responsible for service was performed and an urban/rural description of the municipality or service area provided.

The collection experience expressed as a percentage of paid, unpaid, and gratis calls for all purveyors in the study area who charge a fee-for-service was calculated by tabulating mean responses and the cumulative frequency of responses to a specific question regarding this information. A similar approach was employed to describe the type of requests for service and type of call (emergent or nonemergent patient transport or dry run) that resulted in uncollectable accounts.[a]

---

[a]In analyzing ambulance service costs, we modified the commonly used commercial-municipal-volunteer grouping because we believed a more meaningful comparative cost analysis was possible by using mutually exclusive classes of purveyors based on different financial and staffing patterns. (Appendix 5A contains this typology and definition of terms.)

Analyzing the data was difficult for several reasons. Exact expense records were not maintained. Specific expense items were not accounted for by subcategory but were lumped into general expense accounts. Expenses incurred as a result of the operation of municipal and volunteer services were often not identified in the purveyor's operating statement but were incorporated in a municipal budget. To overcome these obstacles we obtained a description of the item or service for which expenses had been incurred by the purveyor or municipality; consulted with individuals with expertise in insurance coverage, property valuation, and communication services to obtain average cost data; and developed estimates of purveyors' expenses. (Specific approaches to developing estimates for purveyor expenses are described in Appendix 5B.)

In the data collection phase, when requesting summaries of revenue and expenses, it was stressed to all purveyors that information submitted would be held in strict confidence. Furthermore, to enhance cooperation, purveyors were assured that financial data would not be identified by purveyor. This assurance enhanced the prospect of reliable data collection and, in several instances, encouraged purveyors operating in close geographical proximity (and thus in direct competition) to participate in the study. Rather than relying solely on an interview instrument for data collection, when possible we used IRS income tax forms supplied by each purveyor as a check on validity and reliability.

STUDY FINDINGS

Costs Per Run

Among the three general types of purveyors, the mean cost per run for municipals was $46.72; commercials, $33.45; and volunteers, $21.73 (see Tables 5-1, 5-2, and 5-3).

Two methods were used to calculate cost per run. Method I adds all expenses, excluding extreme values, and divides these by the total number of runs by all purveyors in a class. Method II takes the same approach but does not exclude extreme values. We believe Method I may better reflect the underlying cost structure since it cannot be influenced by extremes at either end of a range of values (see Tables 5-4 and 5-5).

Fixed expenses make the most significant contribution to total expenses for all purveyor groups. In relation to total expenses, municipal purveyors have mean fixed expenses of 90 percent; commercial, 84.2 percent; and volunteers, 76 percent. Commercial purveyors, all of whom charge for service, pass these along to the

Table 5-1. Commercial Purveyors: Computation of Costs Per Run[a]

Type A (n=8)				Type B (n=7)			
Purveyor No.	Total Expenses Fiscal Year 1970 (A)	Number of Runs 1970 (B)	Cost Per Run (A) – (B)	Purveyor No.	Total Expenses Fiscal Year 1970 (A)	Number of Runs 1970 (B)	Cost Per Run (A) – (B)
1	$ 70,107	1,740	$40.29	9	$ 40,846	841	$47.00
2	$210,034	5,350	$39.25	10	$ 51,262	1,238	$41.40
3	$ 76,161	1,986	$38.34	11	$139,495	3,756 (PE)	$37.13
4	$ 60,000	1,700	$35.29	12	$ 27,327	750	$36.43
5	$211,765	6,266	$33.79	13	$ 54,039	1,575 (PE)	$34.31
6	$177,285	6,000 (PE)[b]	$29.54	14	$ 44,786	1,379	$32.47
7	$ 84,425	3,383	$26.43	15	$ 4,510	350	$12.88
8	$ 18,833	1,095 (PE)	$17.19[c]				

x = $32.50
S.D. = $7.87
Median = $34.54

x = $34.52
S.D. = $10.69
Median = $36.43

All purveyors (n=15): x = $33.45   S.D. = $9.00   Median = $35.29

[a](See Appendix 5A for an explanation of the typology used in this chapter.)
[b]PE = Purveyor's Estimate.
[c]No salary expense—owner operates service and draws minimal compensation.

Table 5-2. Municipal Purveyors: Computation of Costs Per Run

	Type A (n=8)			Type B (n=2)			Type C (n=6)		
Purveyor No.	Total Expenses FY 1970	Number of Runs 1970	Cost Per Run	Purveyor No.	Total Expenses FY 1970	Number of Runs 1970	Cost Per Run		
1	$ 89,588	661	$135.53	9	$23,572	549	$42.93		
2	$ 29,516	250 (PE)^a	$118.06	10	$ 4,602	269	$17.10		
3	$ 35,586	612	$ 58.14						
4	$ 44,817	1060	$ 42.28						
5	$138,227	3650 (PE)	$ 37.87						
6	$ 7,360	201	$ 36.61						
7	$ 10,550	358	$ 29.46						
8	$ 16,385	885	$ 18.51						

x = $59.56
S.D. = $43.22
Median = $40.88

x = $30.01

	Type C (n=6)		
Purveyor No.	Total Expenses FY 1970	Number of Runs	Cost Per Run
11	$15,533	306	$50.76
12	$ 5,700	120	$47.50
13	$ 7,121	202	$35.25
14	$ 6,700	208	$32.21
15	$ 2,158	75	$28.77
16	$ 978	59*	$16.57

x = $35.18
S.D. = $12.57
Median = $33.73
*Total runs 4/1/70-3/31/71

All Purveyors: n = 16   x = $46.72   S.D. = $33.55   Median = $35.93

^aPE = Purveyor's Estimate.

Table 5-3.   Volunteer Purveyors: Computation of Costs Per Run

	Type A (n=4)				Type B (n=11)		
Purveyor No.	Total Expenses Fiscal Year 1970	Number of Runs 1970	Cost Per Run	Purveyor No.	Total Expenses Fiscal Year 1970	Number of Runs 1970	Cost Per Run
1	$15,640	364	$42.96	5	$3,585	67	$53.50
2	$ 6,450	400	$16.12	6	$8,229	229	$28.18
3	$ 5,540	400	$13.85	7	$4,531	170	$26.65
4	$ 6,688	527	$12.69	8	$7,600	326	$23.31
				9	$7,627	375	$20.33
				10	$6,375	373 (PE)[b]	$17.09
				11	$6,466	380	$17.01
				12	$5,306	319	$16.63
				13	$1,982	120	$16.51
				14	$9,430	614 (PE)	$15.35
				15	$2,250[a]	385	$ 5.84

x = $21.41
S.D. = $14.44
Median = $14.99

x = $21.85
S.D. = $12.12
Median = $17.09

Median = $16.63

All Purveyors: n = 15   x = $21.73   S.D. = $12.23

[a]Purveyor receives large monetary equivalent subsidies.
[b]PE = Purveyor's Estimate.

Table 5-4. Computation of Mean Cost Per Run
Commercial, Municipal, and Volunteer Purveyors—1970

General Classification	Total Expenses All Purveyors	Total Runs All Purveyors	Mean Cost Per Run
Commercial (n=15)	$1,275,875	37,409	$34.11
Municipal (n=16)	$ 438,393	9,465	$46.32
Volunteer (n=15)	$ 97,699	5,112	$19.11

patient. Municipal and volunteer services, while they may make a minimal charge for service and hence recover some expenses from the patient, generally absorb these expenses out of operating funds. For municipal purveyors, operating funds are derived primarily from local taxes; for volunteers, from subscriptions and donations. The high percentage of fixed expenses for all types of purveyors reflects the costs of having vehicles and equipment standing by in readiness to make emergency responses. The substantial expense of standby personnel is incorporated in the fixed expenses of commercial and municipal services.

Costs Per Capita

Costs per capita for the fourteen municipalities studied ranged from $0.43 to $2.90, with a mean of $1.66 and a standard deviation of $0.63 (see Table 5-6). Communities with municipal services had the highest per capita costs due primarily to higher fringe benefits and salaries of ambulance personnel. Even in these communities, the level of these per capita expenditures is significantly below that for other emergency services such as fire and police protection. In one city in the study region served by two commercial purveyors, the annual cost per capita for ambulance service was $1.34 in compari-

Table 5-5. Summary of Mean Costs Per Run Calculated by Method I and Method II for Commercial, Municipal, and Volunteer Purveyors

General Classification	Mean Cost Per Run	
	Method I[a]	Method II[b]
Municipal	$46.72	$46.32
Commercial	$33.45	$34.11
Volunteer	$21.73	$19.11

[a]Calculated as percentage of fixed expenses plus percentage of variable expenses excluding all extreme values and divided by total number of runs by all purveyors in class.
[b]Calculated as total sum of all expenses and divided by total number of runs made by all purveyors in class.

Table 5-6. Calculation of Costs Per Capita: 14 Connecticut Cities and Towns—1970

Town, City, or Service Area	Urban/Rural Classification	Type and Number of Purveyors	Total Cost of Operation: Adjusted	1970 Census	Cost Per Capita
New Britain	Urban	(1) Municipal Type A (1) Commercial Type A	$198,227	83,441	$2.38
Meriden	Urban	(2) Commercial Type B	$ 74,827	55,959	$1.34
Milford	Urban	(1) Commercial Type B	$ 93,401	50,858	$1.87
Middletown	Urban	(2) Commercial		36,924	
Middlefield	Rural	(1) Type A		4,132	
Portland	Urban (part)	(1) Type B		8,812	
Haddam	Rural			4,934	
Middletown Region			$ 77,900	54,802	$1.42
Newington	Urban (part)	(1) Volunteer Type B	$ 11,100	26,037	$ .43
Plainville	Urban (part)	(1) Municipal Type A	$ 35,886	16,733	$2.14
Southington	Urban (part)	(1) Municipal Type A	$ 89,888	30,946	$2.90
Wallingford	Urban (part)	(1) Municipal Type A	$ 44,817	35,714	$1.26
Berlin-Kensington	Urban (part)	(1) Municipal Type A (1) Volunteer Type B	$ 33,466	14,149	$2.37
Cromwell	Urban (part)	(1) Municipal Type C	$ 5,700[a]	7,400	$ .77
Deep River	Rural	(1) Volunteer Type B	$ 5,131	3,690	$1.39

n = 11
x = $1.66 per capita
S.D. = $0.63

[a]Purveyor received substantial vehicle subsidy.

son to $24.82 for police service and $18.78 for fire service in fiscal 1970–71.

Patterns of Service

All ambulance purveyors in the study region provided both emergency and nonemergency service. In a subsample, 13,063 trips were made by fourteen purveyors. Of these, 62 percent (n=8,121) were emergency responses and 38 percent (n=4,492) were for reasons of nonurgent patient transportation. These data are consistent with the patterns of service for Connecticut described in Chapter 3.

Collection Experience

The collection experience of purveyors who charge for service reveals that a mean of 22 percent of these ambulance runs were not paid for in 1970. Fifty percent of all ambulance purveyors identified the prime source of unpaid runs as nonresidents requiring emergency service. While poor records do not permit a conclusive statement based on service characteristics, it appears that a substantial number of these unpaid accounts are traffic-accident victims.

Subsidies

Approximately one-fifth of all purveyors in Connecticut received fixed or variable-sum monetary subsidies in 1970, and approximately one-third reported some form of monetary-equivalent subsidization. Monetary subsidies were usually received by commercial and volunteer purveyors, while monetary-equivalent subsidies were received primarily by volunteer and municipal services. The grant of a monetary subsidy to a commercial purveyor has the effect of increasing net receipts.[3]

In Connecticut, monetary subsidies are usually granted by a local government based on two considerations: the need to provide emergency ambulance service to local residents and the recognition of the potential uncollectibility of charges made for service. Monetary subsidies received by volunteer purveyors help to defray operating expenses and are granted because of the public-service nature of ambulance service.

Monetary-equivalent subsidies received by volunteer and municipal purveyors have the effect of reducing operating expenses and/or eliminating the need for certain sizable capital expenditures out of operating funds for items essential to providing adequate service. As an example, one Connecticut volunteer fire department purveyor reported that total expenses in fiscal 1970 were $2,250—$5.84 per run for 385 runs. This purveyor was heavily subsidized by the local municipal government and a private foundation. Heated garage space; use of the police department's central dispatch service; and gas, oil, and maintenance were all provided by the municipal government. A private foundation aided the purveyor in a vehicle purchase with a $3,200 grant. Had subsidies from both sources not been forthcoming, approximately $4,600 would have been added to the expense of operations, thus raising the total operating expense figure to $6,850 or $17.79 per run. For all purveyors receiving monetary-equivalent subsidies, no conditions of eligibility aside from continued existence of service were in effect.

In several interviews, purveyors mentioned that a significant problem occurs in caring for Medicaid recipients. Frequently, these individuals have no way of getting to the hospital for minor ailments, except by ambulance. In most communities, Medicaid will pay for an ambulance trip but not for a taxi or bus. Often this ties up an ambulance for long periods of time because the patient must be transported back home after treatment if a physician certifies that this is necessary, and physicians will rarely deny such transport to a patient. Using emergency ambulance service for routine transport may endanger others who might need emergency service. The issue of Medicare and Medicaid reimbursement for emergency and routine ambulance service was beyond the scope of this study.[4]

SUMMARY OF FINDINGS

Because of the difficulty in obtaining ambulance cost data, we focused most of our analysis on one fourteen-town area which was representative of the state and which contained unusually reliable data. In this area, the mean cost per ambulance run was $46.72 for municipal, $33.45 for commercial, and $21.73 for volunteer purveyors. The higher municipal costs primarily reflect more generous salaries and fringe benefits for ambulance personnel while the lower volunteer costs primarily reflect considerable donated ambulance personnel time.

Costs per capita for ambulance services averaged less than $2 per year compared with about $25 for police protection and about $19 for fire services. Of the purveyors who charge for service, over 20 percent of ambulance runs are not paid for by the user. Approximately 20 percent of all purveyors receive some type of monetary subsidy and approximately one-third receive some form of monetary-equivalent subsidy. While upgrading components of ambulance services (e.g., vehicles, equipment, and personnel) will increase service costs, they will still remain significantly below costs for police and fire services.

Appendix 5A

Typology and Definition of Terms

A. AMBULANCE PURVEYOR TYPOLOGY

Commercial Purveyor: an ambulance service that is privately owned or incorporated and operated for the purpose of making a profit.

Type A Commercial Purveyor: a commercial firm whose sole business activity is the provision of ambulance service.

Type B Commercial Purveyor: an ambulance firm that provides ambulance service in conjunction with other business activities.

Municipal Purveyor: an ambulance service for which the primary source of financial support (> 50%) is from local taxes.

Type A Municipal Purveyor: a municipal ambulance service staffed only by full-time paid personnel.

Type B Municipal Purveyor: a municipal ambulance service staffed by both full-time paid personnel and volunteers.

Type C Municipal Purveyor: a municipal ambulance service staffed only by volunteers.

Volunteer Purveyor: an ambulance service for which the primary source of financial support (> 50%) is from donations and/or local subscriptions.

Type A Volunteer Purveyor: a volunteer ambulance service staffed by some paid personnel who receive minimal remuneration.

Type B Volunteer Purveyor: a voluntary ambulance service staffed by nonpaid personnel.

Hospital-Based Purveyor: an ambulance service owned and operated by a hospital, supported by fees for service and/or institutional operating funds, and staffed by hospital personnel.

B. DEFINITION OF TERMS

Variable Costs: costs that vary directly and proportionately with the volume of ambulance runs (e.g., the amount of service provided).

Fixed or Nonvariable Costs: costs that do not vary with volume (or the level of service rendered) but are incurred with the passage of time independent of the level of activity.

Expenses: the cost incurred in connection with the earning of revenue, incurred but not necessarily paid (consumed) in a given period of time.[a]

Expenditure: that which occurs when an asset or service is acquired, and may be made by cash, exchange of another asset, or by incurring a liability. It is incurred and paid (consumed) in a given period of time.

Summary of Revenue and Expenses: for commercial purveyors, an accounting report similar to an income statement that summarizes the revenue items, the expense items, and the difference between them (net income) for an accounting period; for municipal and volunteer purveyors, a statement of financial operations that summarizes expenditures and the amount of financial support and revenue, if any, received for a specified period.

Cash Basis of Accounting: a practice not in accordance with generally accepted accounting principles but allowed by the U.S. Internal Revenue Service (IRS) for income tax purposes whereby revenue is recognized only when cash is received.

Accrual Concept of Accounting: an accounting concept (often described as the matching concept) where expenses recognized in an accounting period are matched with the revenues recognized in that period.

Subsidy to Commercial Purveyor: a guarantee of revenue to a purveyor on either a fixed or variable basis, with or without conditions, from a government or nongovernment source; or receipt of a monetary equivalent in goods and services for which the purveyor incurs no or token expense.

[a]The terms "expense" and "expenditure" are sometimes used interchangeably, particularly when the cash basis of accounting is used. Such a distinction is important, however, when the accrual concept of accounting is used.

Subsidy to Municipal Purveyor: a monetary contribution to the municipal purveyor on either a fixed or variable basis, with or without conditions, from the state or federal government or from private sources (including private citizens, civic organizations, and private business enterprises) whose economic base is not from local taxes; or receipt of a monetary equivalent in free goods and services from the state or federal government or from private sources for which the municipal purveyor incurs no or token expense. This subsidy excludes small monetary donations solicited and/or accepted from the general public and includes monetary equivalents from private citizens.

Subsidy to Volunteer Purveyor: a monetary contribution to a volunteer ambulance organization on either a fixed or variable basis, with or without conditions, from a government or nongovernment source; or receipt of a monetary equivalent in free goods and services from a government or nongovernment source for which the volunteer organization incurs no or token expense. This subsidy excludes supporting donations and subscriptions of $100 or less from citizens benefiting from the service provided by the volunteer purveyor as well as donated time by members of the volunteer organization or others acting as private citizens.

Subsidy to Hospital Purveyor: a guarantee of revenue to the ambulance service of a hospital on either a fixed or variable basis, with or without conditions, from a government or nongovernment source; or receipt of a monetary equivalent in free goods and services for which the ambulance service incurs no or token expense.

Fixed Monetary Subsidy: a fixed monetary amount granted to a purveyor for a specified period (e.g., per annum) and unrelated to the number of runs made during that period.

Variable-Sum Monetary Subsidy: a monetary subsidy granted to a purveyor based on a certain dollar amount over a specified period of time, related to the number of runs made during that period.

Appendix 5B

Approaches to the Development of Ambulance Cost Estimates

Cost of Insurance: Information on annual rates for both vehicle and professional liability insurance for varying limits of liability for purveyors operating in both urban and rural areas was requested from at least three of the primary ambulance insurers in the area. The vehicle insurance policy included bodily injury, property damage, comprehensive, and collision (with deductible) provisions. The firms were asked to quote rates on comprehensive and collision provisions for a specific type of ambulance. Professional liability insurance rates should be requested on a per-vehicle basis for at least $100,000/$300,000 limits of coverage. Estimates of the total cost of insurance for a specific purveyor who cannot provide that information were derived by matching the response to a question in a composite questionnaire requesting information on the types and levels of coverage with the appropriate rate quotations obtained from insurers.

Cost of Physical Plant: In developing an estimate of the overhead expense of providing garage space for vehicles, a firm with considerable experience in commercial real estate management in the study area was consulted. This firm was asked to provide the typical overhead costs per month for keeping one vehicle in a heated garage based on varying types of buildings located in the study area. Estimates of such overhead costs per month for an urban area of Connecticut in 1971 were:

Municipal building (brick): $50
Firehouse (brick): $40–50
Separate vehicle garage (heated): $30
Private resident-type garage (unheated): $15

Cost of Fringe Benefits: Fire and police department personnel staffing municipal ambulance services receive considerable fringe benefits as a result of their status as municipal employees, unlike personnel staffing commercial and volunteer ambulance service. A full fringe-benefit package includes pensions, survivor benefits, health insurance, life insurance, and workmen's compensation. These benefits are received over and above gross salary. A reasonable estimate of the cost of operations of a municipal ambulance service must take into account the full cost of such fringe benefits. One method of determining this is to ask the director of finance of a town within the study area. In Connecticut, 35 percent of gross salary expense was a conservative estimate of the cost of providing a full benefit package including all the items mentioned above.

Cost of Communication Services: The average annual cost of shared communication services for ambulance purveyors in the study area was determined from telephone company representatives and shared operating communication stations. Data collected for the Connecticut study revealed that $180 per year for a shared telephone answering service and $300 per year for shared central dispatching service are reasonable rough estimates.

Depreciation Expense: If purveyors depreciate vehicles and equipment but cannot provide an exact depreciation expense figure, a reasonable estimate can be made by employing IRS guidelines in an acceptable and conservative manner. The useful life of an ambulance vehicle included in the IRS category of "Automobiles: Passenger— Used by Commercial Enterprises Other Than Public Utility" is five years under the provisions of Depreciation Bulletin F (Revised 1942) and four years or less under revised Procedures 62-21. Bulletin F guidelines, however, remain acceptable to the IRS. Selecting the five-year useful–life guideline and employing a straight-line depreciation method, ambulance vehicle depreciation can be calculated on the basis of initial cost. Depreciation was only credited to the purveyor if the age of the vehicle was five years or less.

A number of municipal and volunteer purveyors do not depreciate vehicles and equipment and thus show no corresponding expense item. If the vehicles and equipment had been purchased out of operating or capital funds, the purchase cost of the asset could be allocated over the useful life of the vehicle—hence an expense category of "Annual Allocation of the Initial Cost of Vehicle Assets" can be created arbitrarily. The purpose of establishing this expense category is to account for the expenditure for the vehicle over a period of time rather than only in the year of acquisition. This item is not to be construed as depreciation, although the method of estimating it is the same.

Fundamental to performing a comparative analysis of the financial operations of ambulance purveyors is the establishment of a uniform chart of accounts. In Connecticut and probably elsewhere in the United States, financial statements lack such uniformity. Statements not submitted on the revenue and expense form provided as part of an interview instrument may vary in format and the manner in which expenses and revenues are itemized. For the purpose of undertaking a comparison of costs per trip and a percentage of fixed and variable costs among types of purveyors, it was necessary to construct a list of expense groupings into which the various expense items incurred by purveyors can be posted logically. It should be reiterated at this point that the terms "expense" and "expenditure" were used interchangeably since our analysis was based on the cash-flow method of accounting that seems to predominate among ambulance purveyors. The following is a suggested format of cost analysis identifying the expense groupings and individual items of expense that are incorporated in each:

FIXED EXPENSES

Direct salary expense: driver and attendant wages
Support salary expense: clerical and managerial salary compensation to officers
Fringe Benefits: workmen's compensation, health and life insurance, and pension payments
Depreciation of ambulance vehicles and equipment: depreciation expense for vehicles and equipment
(or)
Annual allocation of initial cost of vehicle assets: estimated allocation of cost of vehicle asset for current fiscal year
Insurance: vehicle, professional liability, and business
Overhead on physical plant: utilities, building depreciation, maintenance, property taxes, and rent
Professional fees: legal, accounting, and collection expenses

Office operation expense: office supplies, telephone, and office and
   equipment depreciation
Communication expense: rental of communications equipment and
   fees paid for answering service and central dispatching service
Other fixed expenses: public relations, travel, dues, licenses, taxes

VARIABLE EXPENSES

Vehicle operation and maintenance: gas, oil, regular maintenance,
   and minor repairs
Other variable expenses: laundry, linen, and over-the-road expense

✳ *Part III*

The Hospital Phase

✳ *Chapter 6*

Hospital Emergency Departments

INTRODUCTION AND OBJECTIVES

In many parts of the United States the hospital emergency department (ED) stands alone as the one continuously available point of access for patients seeking medical care. It is the institutional focal point for treating a myriad of problems ranging from the simple to the severe. Hospital emergency departments in the United States have experienced an annual growth of 36 percent in patient visits between 1966 and 1973, a rate unmatched by any other area of the hospital.[1] EDs are often described as poorly organized and are accused of providing fragmented, episodic, low-quality patient care at an unacceptably high cost.[2] In defense of EDs, only recently have they received adequate medical and administrative attention, support, and budget. And most emergency departments provide care to patients with nonurgent problems as well as to those who are critically ill.[3]

The enormous increase in the number of emergency department visits cannot be attributed solely to population growth, increasing numbers of accidents or changes in third party reimbursement. The increase also represents a shifting pattern in medical care organization. As early as 1961, it was reported that the function and responsibility of the emergency department has changed, ". . . what was once the accident room designed to handle acute emergency patients in trauma is now regarded, at least by the general public, as the appropriate initial source of medical care for a wide variety of medical, surgical, pediatric and even psychiatric problems."[4]

The emergency department can fill a number of roles: (1) an acute care center where the seriously injured and critically ill patient is brought for immediate medical and surgical care; (2) a back-up medical facility for patients unable or unwilling to contact their own physician; (3) a primary care center for patients without their own physician; and (4) a physician's workshop.[5]

In 1974, there were 1,127,000 visits to thirty-four hospital emergency departments in Connecticut.[6] This represents an increase of 262 percent since 1960, with the greatest increase occurring since 1965 and in the rural areas of the state. Emergency-service utilization has far outstripped population growth, which has increased by only 18 percent since 1960. Moreover, emergency department admissions to the hospital now comprise almost one-third of total hospital admissions in Connecticut. These figures reflect the increasing importance of the emergency department to hospital operations.

Recognizing the increased volume and complexity of problems confronting today's hospital emergency department, this chapter begins with a discussion of categorization as a mechanism for rationalizing hospital emergency resources. We then present an evaluation of Connecticut's ED capabilities through an examination of four of its elements: physical plant, equipment, primary and support staff, and administration. We also examine hospital services which support Connecticut EDs and assess the state's disaster planning capabilities.

In evaluating the capabilities of Connecticut EDs, we are relying on input data. Our inventory of ED elements will be compared to professionally mandated standards, and represents the first step toward the development of a categorization plan for the state's hospital emergency departments.

CATEGORIZATION OF HOSPITAL EMERGENCY DEPARTMENTS

While all EDs must meet certain minimum criteria, to upgrade all departments so that they possess optimal capabilities would require significant investment in renovation and equipment and increased staffing by personnel trained in critical care techniques. This alternative is economically unsound and is not necessary to provide high quality emergency care. Just as every institution should not attempt to offer open heart surgery or high energy radiation therapy, all hospitals should not attempt to provide the most comprehensive emergency services.

A more feasible approach would be to upgrade all EDs to an accepted minimal level and to categorize them according to their level of capability. Categorization would have such advantages as:

1. Helping to ensure the adequate delivery of emergency care of the type and complexity needed
2. Reducing the total cost for the provision of emergency medical services in a community or region
3. Conserving scarce health manpower resources and ensuring that each individual performs the job for which he or she is properly trained
4. Strengthening nonemergency care services in a community or region.

To date, two basic approaches to categorization have been proposed.[7] One, which we term structural categorization, classifies hospital emergency-care capabilities according to the degree of comprehensiveness of the services. Another, which we term problem-specific categorization, classifies hospital emergency departments according to their ability to treat certain kinds of emergencies. Both categorization schemes imply a regional focus which requires coordination of existing hospital facilities, manpower, and equipment resources in a geographic area. This in turn demands cooperative arrangements between hospitals, physicians, ambulance purveyors, and police and fire departments for dealing with different types of emergencies.

Both the structural and problem-specific categorization schemes are developed around a set of what is commonly termed inventory criteria as distinct from performance criteria.[8] Inventory criteria address quantities of emergency response capabilities while performance criteria are based on clinical indicators which include the quality as well as the quantity of emergency response capabilities. While performance criteria have clear advantages over inventory criteria, they are presently only in the developmental stage.[9]

The structural approach is the backbone of the American Medical Association's (AMA's) categorization scheme which defines four categories of hospital emergency services.[10] These categories and the scope of capabilities required for each are:

1. *Comprehensive Emergency Service:* The hospital should be fully equipped, prepared, and staffed to provide prompt, complete, and advanced medical care for all emergencies, including those requiring the most complex and specialized services for newborn infants and children. It should have a capacity of providing

consultative support to professional personnel of other hospitals
and health facilities in the same region.

2. *Major Emergency Service:* The hospital should be equipped, prepared, and staffed in all medical and surgical specialties to render
resuscitation and life support for adults, children, and newborn
infants. It should also supply definitive care for all such patients,
except for the occasional patient who requires follow-through
care in very specialized units. Transfer may be necessary and
should be under prior agreement with other hospitals.

3. *General Emergency Service:* The hospital should be equipped,
prepared, and staffed in the medical and surgical specialties
necessary to render resuscitative and life-support care of persons
of all ages who are critically ill or injured. The availability of sup-
plementary specialty services should be prearranged with non-
staff specialists. Transfer of patients for specialty care should be
made by prior agreement with other hospitals.

4. *Basic Emergency Service:* The hospital should be equipped, prepared, and adequately staffed to render emergency resuscitative
and life-support medical services for patients of all ages. Transfer
when necessary should be under prior agreement with other
hospitals.

Another example of structural categorization is the Hospital Council
of Southern California (HCSC) plan.[11]

In recent years, EMS planning activities in the United States have
emphaszied structural categorization. But these plans fail to consider
differences in the diagnostic-specific case mix of emergencies by type
or frequency of occurrence. Six types of emergencies have been dis-
tinguished by some health-planning authorities:[12]

1. Trauma and acute surgical problems
2. Cardiac emergencies
3. Psychiatric emergencies
4. High-risk neonatal and pediatric cases
5. Poisonings
6. Drug and alcohol overdoses.

Each of these emergencies will require a special response. For example, Shan Cretin has shown that certain cardiac emergencies are
more time-dependent than other types of emergencies.[13] The cardiac
patient should benefit by being taken directly to the nearest emergency facility for diagnosis, stabilization, and life support. On the
other hand, some psychiatric emergencies might be adequately

stabilized by an emergency medical technician (EMT) in the ambulance and then brought to the appropriate psychiatric facility, perhaps bypassing the nearest hospital. The problem-specific approach begins to take into account the varying requirements for life support and definitive treatment presented by different emergency problems.

One problem-specific categorization scheme defines four levels of care capabilities for each of the six diagnostic categories of emergencies listed above.[14] These levels are:

1. Treatment of all cases
2. Treatment of all but the most serious cases
3. Provision of only basic stabilization and immediate transfer
4. No capability in the diagnostic area.

HOSPITAL EMERGENCY DEPARTMENT CAPABILITIES

Prior to 1972, little was known about the thirty-five Connecticut hospital emergency departments in terms of their basic medical capacity or organizational structure. In order to upgrade all Connecticut EDs to accepted minimum levels and to provide the information necessary for implementing a statewide categorization scheme, certain data are needed.

We focused our study on Connecticut's thirty-five short-term acute general hospital EDs. Although other medical-care institutions in the state provide some emergency service (e.g., two Veterans Administration hospitals, state mental institutions, industrial clinics, and three group health plans), these facilities treat a limited population. They are valuable community resources and should be included when developing disaster or other contingency plans but they were not considered primary providers of emergency medical care because of their limited access by the public.

While aware that all thirty-five hospitals could not and should not meet the highest level of ED capability, data concerning Connecticut EDs were compared to the following guidelines, which in our opinion were the most useful:

Professional Organization	*Descriptive Title*
American College of Surgeons (ACS) Committee on Trauma	Comprehensive emergency service
American Medical Association (AMA)	Comprehensive emergency service
Hospital Council of Southern California (HCSC)	Comprehensive 24-hour emergency service
Joint Commission on Accreditation of Hospitals (JCAH)	Standards for accreditation

While emergency departments vary in size, capability, and objectives, four elements are common to all: physical plant, equipment, staff, and administration. We will review each of these elements, as well as those services that directly support ED functions (blood bank, clinical laboratories, and radiology) and those that provide backup to the ED patient (the intensive-care unit, the coronary-care unit, and the operating room).

Physical Plant

Our examination of ED physical plants included a review of four subelements: pedestrian and vehicular access, the presence of designated patient care areas, staff work areas, and family and patient waiting areas. Easy pedestrian and vehicular access requires that the ED entrance be direct to the outside, be at ground level, and be clearly marked. Each member of the survey team noted whether one could locate the emergency department without difficulty and if the entrance was clearly marked. As presented in Table 6-1, 80 percent of the emergency departments were rated as having a clearly marked entrance. All had a separate outside entrance and all but one was located at ground level.

With regard to designated patient care areas, the Joint Commission on Accreditation of Hospitals (JCAH) recommends examination and treatment rooms, a minor surgery area, and a plaster room. All thirty-five emergency departments have each of these. One standard mentioned by the JCAH and recommended by the American College of Surgeons (ACS) calls for the separation of the critically ill or injured patient from less seriously ill patients.[15] This standard is met by 80 percent of Connecticut EDs (see Table 6-1).

The presence of observation beds in the emergency department permits greater flexibility of care. For example, a physician can observe a patient, who presents a difficult diagnostic problem, in the ED without occupying an inpatient bed or emergency care area and thus help prevent unnecessary hospital admissions. Only 40 percent of Connecticut hospital EDs have observation areas.

The presence of a designated area for press, police, and ambulance attendants could enhance relations with these agencies and serve to keep individuals away from hospital staff work areas. Only 29 percent of the emergency departments in Connecticut have this designated area. By having a quiet area removed from the main patient waiting room, the family of a critical patient is allowed privacy and a place where physicians are able to communicate without disturbance. Table 6-1 shows that only 37 percent of the emergency departments have provided space for a "quiet room."

**Table 6-1. Physical Plant Recommended Criteria for Emergency Departments
How Connecticut Hospitals Measure Up to Professional Standards**

	Recommended By:				Emergency Departments in Connecticut	
Physical Plant Criteria	The American College of Surgeons	The American Medical Association	Hospital Council Southern California	JCAH	#	%
open 24 hours a day	X	X	X	X	35	100
separate outside entrance	X	X	X	X	35	100
registration area	X			X	35	100
examination and treatment rooms	X	X	X	X	35	100
minor surgery	X	X	X	X	35	100
plaster room	X		X	X	35	100
observation area	X		X	X	14	40
patient waiting area	X		X		35	100
physician's and nurse's work area	X		X		35	100
supplemental power provisions					34	97
ground level entrance	X	X			32	91
overhead coverage for ambulance unloading area		X			28	80
clearly marked entrance	X	X			28	80
separation of critically ill patients	X			X	28	80
adequate storage area	X				28	80
doctors on-call room in the emergency service	X				13	37
quiet room					12	34
separate ambulance entrance						
press, police, and ambulance attendants area	X				7	20

Table 6-2. Emergency Departments in Connecticut Age and Plans for Overhaul

Year Built	Number	Number Planning Overhaul	Percent
Before 1950	11	11	100
1951–1960	8	7	88
1961–1965	5	1	20
1966–1970	4	1	25
Since 1970	7	1	14
Total	35	21	60

Additional factors to be considered when assessing the adequacy of an emergency department facility are: its age, whether or not new construction or overhaul is planned, and when the last overhaul took place. Table 6-2 displays the age of Connecticut emergency departments and plans for their overhaul.

As seen in Table 6-2, 53 percent of the ED facilities were built prior to 1960. But 85 percent of those emergency departments are planning new construction or overhaul.

Equipment

The American College of Surgeons lists a minimum of nine equipment items as essential to the emergency department. Table 6-3 presents a checklist of these items and their recommended location. A cardiac defibrillator, tracheal intubation equipment, and a prepared poison tray are especially important. The availability of a defibrillator in the emergency department is imperative because any loss of time in treating a patient in cardiac standstill or ventricular fibrillation could result in the patient's demise. Only twenty-nine hospitals indicate that a defibrillator is available in the ED at all times. Table 6-3 reveals that some emergency departments have interpreted the recommendations of the JCAH loosely, and consider themselves adequately equipped if these items are available to, but not necessarily present in, the emergency department.

A top priority in the management of the multiple-trauma patient is the establishment and maintenance of an adequate airway. The trauma patient suffering from airway obstruction will often require immediate endotracheal intubation. Two hospitals reported not having endotracheal intubation trays available in the ED.

While it is not essential or even desirable for each hospital to be a poison control center, it is essential that there be a prepared poison tray in the emergency department at all times. Although the degree

Table 6-3. Resuscitation Equipment Recommended Criteria for Emergency Departments How Connecticut Hospitals Measure Up to Professional Standards

Equipment Criteria	The American College of Surgeons	The American Medical Association	Hospital Council Southern California	JCAH	Emergency Departments in Connecticut #	Emergency Departments in Connecticut %
wall or portable oxygen	X		X	X	35	100
wall or portable suction	X	X	X	X	35	100
endotracheal intubation equipment in the emergency department	X	X	X	X	33	94
poison tray in the emergency department	X	X	X	X	32	91
ECG in the emergency department 24 hours a day	X	X			27	77
cardioscope in the emergency department 24 hours a day	X	X			28	80
defibrillator in the emergency department 24 hours a day	X	X			29	83
thoractemy equipment in the emergency department	X	X			28	80
venous pressure sets in the emergency department	X	X			32	91

Table 6-4.   Availability of Prepared Emergency Trays in Connecticut Emergency Departments

	Available in Hospital Emergency Department	
Prepared Emergency Tray	Number	Percent
Lumbar Puncture	31	88
Paracentesis	31	88
Thoracentesis	28	80
Venous Pressure	32	91
Suture Sets	35	100

of sophistication and the amount of equipment may vary, this tray should contain at least: a list of antidotes for specific poisons, stomach tubes, syringes, and oral airways.[16] The location of this tray in another part of the hospital can result in unnecessary delay and might further complicate a patient's condition. Three Connecticut emergency departments are deficient here.

The availability of other specially prepared emergency "trays" was examined. Table 6-4 shows that most but not all emergency departments have these trays.

Primary and Support Staff

While physical plant and equipment are major determinants of good emergency department function, the most important element is personnel. The JCAH states: "Service must be available 24 hours a day, and medical staff coverage must be adequate to ensure that an applicant for treatment will be seen within a reasonable length of time relative to his illness or injury. . . ." There should be an adequate number of nurses for the amount and type of care to be provided.[17]

Some hospitals interpret the commission's standards to allow staff to have other responsibilities while working in the emergency department. Table 6-5 shows that in four hospitals, the first call physician is not required to be in the emergency department twenty-four hours a day. This also holds for nursing personnel where eleven hospitals do not require the presence of nursing personnel in the ED around the clock. Considering that an emergency patient is often brought in without any warning and can arrive at any time of day or night, some health professional trained in all aspects of acute patient management must always be present in the ED. Unless a nurse practitioner or physician's associate has been thoroughly trained in these techniques, a physician will be required.

Table 6-5. Primary and Support Staff
Recommended Criteria for Emergency Departments
How Connecticut Hospitals Measure Up to Professional Standards

Staff Criteria	Recommended By:				Emergency Departments in Connecticut	
	The American College of Surgeons	The American Medical Association	Hospital Council Southern California	JCAH	#	%
physician coverage in the emergency department 24 hours a day (no additional hospital duties)	X	X			31	88
nursing coverage 24 hours a day in the emergency department (no additional duties)	X	X			24	69
24 hour a day availability of specialty consultation:						
general surgery	X	X	X		35	100
internal medicine	X	X	X		35	100
obstetrics and gynecology	X	X	X		35	100
pediatrics	X	X	X		34	97
radiology	X	X	X		33	94
orthopedics	X	X	X		33	94
anesthesiology	X	X	X		33	94
cardiology	X	X	X		32	91
ear, nose, and throat	X	X	X		32	91
psychiatry	X	X	X		31	89
plastic surgery	X	X	X		25	71
neurosurgery	X	X	X		25	71
neurology	X	X	X		21	68
all of the above					14	40

Chapter 7 offers an analysis of medical specialty consultation to EDs and this issue will not be reviewed here. The accessibility of physician specialists will be a major factor in determining what levels of care each emergency department can provide and such information will be essential for any categorization plan. Table 6–5 reveals that fourteen hospitals (40 percent) have around-the-clock access to all types of medical specialties.

Three inhospital capabilities which provide critical support to the emergency care rendered in the ED are: renal or peritoneal dialysis—for the treatment of drug ingestion; cardiopulmonary by-pass—for the treatment of chest injuries; neurosurgery—for the treatment of acute head and spinal cord injuries.

While these capabilities are rarely part of the patient's immediate ED care, their presence is often lifesaving and can obviate the transfer of patients to another medical facility. These capabilities will also be major determinants in any EMS categorization scheme. Table 6–6 displays the availability of these services by region.

Administration

Because of the increasing complexity of patient care demands, the provision of emergency medical care often requires integration and cooperation of many medical services, including: medicine, surgery, pediatrics, obstetrics and gynecology, and psychiatry. Paralleling this multidisciplinary involvement in patient care is a need for multidisciplinary administrative organization. Because each professional service requires different types of support facilities, services, and equipment, it is logical that each of these disciplines be included in the coordination and supervision of emergency care activities. Consequently, emergency departments might best be guided by a representative committee composed of medical staff, nursing, and administration. Table 6–7 reveals that twenty-seven emergency departments have an EMS committee but that only sixteen of these have representatives from the medical staff, nursing, and administration.

Because of its increasing importance in the health care system, the emergency service can no longer be considered as the stepchild of the hospital's inpatient functions, but should be given the recognition and support needed to fulfill its mission. The Joint Commission standards state: "When warranted by its activities and its degree of complexity, the emergency service should be organized as a department."[18] The American College of Surgeons (ACS) Committee on Trauma concurs.[19] Only twenty Connecticut emergency services (57 percent) have departmental status. (The term "emergency depart-

Table 6–6. Availability of Renal or Peritoneal Dialysis, Cardiopulmonary By-Pass, and Neurosurgical Capabilities, by Region

Region	Number of Hospitals	Dialysis		By-Pass		Neurosurgeons	
		Number	Percent	Number	Percent	Number	Percent
S. Central	6	4	66	3	50	5	83
Capital	10	4	40	3	50	7	70
S. West	4	3	75	0	—	4	100
Bridgeport	3	2	66	1	33	3	100
Waterbury	2	1	50	0	—	2	100
Middletown	1	0	—	0	—	0	—
S. East	2	0	—	1	50	2	100
N. West	3	0	—	1	33	0	—
N. East	2	2	100	0	—	0	—
Danbury	2	1	50	1	50	1	50
Total	35	17	48	10	20	24	69

Table 6-7.   Administrative Organization
Recommended Criteria for Emergency Departments
How Connecticut Hospitals Measure Up to Professional Standards

Administrative Criteria	Recommended By:				Emergency Departments in Connecticut	
	The American College of Surgeons	The American Medical Association	Hospital Council Southern California	JCAH	#	%
emergency department guided by general written policies	X	X	X	X	35	100
emergency department committee	X		X	X	27	77
emergency department as a separate hospital department	X	X		X	20	57
Specific written policies regarding:						
communications with a poison control center		X		X	30	85
defined scope of treatment allowed in the emergency department				X	29	83
notification of a patient's private physician				X	27	77
transfer of patients to other health care facilities				X	25	71

management of the alcoholic and drug addict		X	25	71
communications with other health agencies, e.g., health department		X	24	68
methods for the procurement of equipment and medications		X	22	63
job descriptions		X	20	57
utilization of observation beds		X	10^a	70
medical records maintained on all patients	X	X	35	100
on-going record review	X	X	23	66
emergency department record incorporated in the patient's total hospital record		X	17	49

[a] n=14 emergency departments with observation beds.

ment" is used throughout this book even though true departmental status does not exist in all Connecticut hospitals.)

Because of the lifesaving implications of the actions of ED personnel, the presence of ED guidelines is useful for adequate guidance of professional activities. According to the JCAH: "There should be written policies concerning the extent of treatment to be carried out in the emergency service. Such policies must be approved by the medical staff and by the hospital management."[20]

All ED written policies and procedures were reviewed by the survey team. A checklist of eleven items recommended by the Joint Commission and the American College of Surgeons served as a yardstick. Table 6-7 reveals a number of deficiencies regarding written policies.

Concerning ED medical records, the Joint Commission states:

> A medical record shall be kept for every patient receiving emergency service; it shall become an official hospital record. . . . A review of emergency room records shall be conducted regularly to evaluate the quality of emergency medical care. . . . It is desirable that the patient's emergency record be incorporated in his previous hospital chart. . . .[21]

All Connecticut emergency departments maintain medical records on all patients (Table 6-7).

For effective emergency care a complete medical record must be maintained and be immediately available to the physician in the emergency department. An immediately accessible record permits the physician to review the patient's past medical history, hospital records, and any other factors that might assist in diagnosis, treatment, and management (e.g, allergic reactions). The ACS, Committee on Trauma, recommends that every patient should have a permanent record containing the history, findings, and treatment, or disposition,[22] while the JCAH suggests that "it is desirable that the patient's emergency record be incorporated in his previous hospital record."[23] Table 6-7 shows that a significant number of Connecticut EDs do not maintain a complete hospital record which includes the ED visit.

Medical records should be reviewed periodically to help assess the quality of care being provided. Regular review provides information concerning the quality of care being provided in the emergency department and serves as a data base for providing new services, augmenting staff, and planning new systems. Regular review also provides an educational vehicle for physicians and other health personnel. The American Medical Association recommends that all emergency services (regardless of the level of care they provide) should conduct an ongoing review of patient records: "Audits and reviews shall be made of the emergency department services in the same manner as for other departments of the hospital. This shall include periodic morbidity reviews."[24] The JCAH also requires that "a review of emergency room records shall be conducted regularly to evaluate the quality of emergency medical care."[25] In Connecticut, only two-thirds of the hospitals conduct an on-going review of emergency department records (see Table 6–7).

ESSENTIAL SUPPORT SERVICES
FOR THE EMERGENCY DEPARTMENT

The availability of certain essential support services were also reviewed. These include: the blood bank, X-ray, and the clinical laboratory. The JCAH requires that radiologic and clinical laboratory facilities "be readily available for use at all times."[26]

While all hospitals in Connecticut maintain clinical laboratories, not enough data were gathered to determine the twenty-four-hour availability of service. Information was obtained on laboratory facilities located in the emergency department. Table 6–8 reveals that all but one hospital has complete X-ray facilities including angiography available around the clock.

All hospitals maintain a blood bank; however, only three-quarters of hospitals have a blood bank in operation around the clock. All hospitals reported the blood bank technicians are on-call twenty-four hours a day to respond to an emergency.

The American College of Surgeons recommends that separate laboratory and X-ray facilities be located in the emergency department.[27] Only six emergency departments maintain their own X-ray facilities and only two have their own laboratory facilities (see Table 6–8). While these units may reduce transportation and waiting time, their absence is probably not critical if the ED has easy, twenty-four-hour access to the hospital facility.

We examined the availability of special hospital support services such as intensive care units, coronary care units, operating rooms, and postoperative recovery areas. In recent years, heavy emphasis has been placed on the need for special units which are designed, staffed, and equipped to provide highly skilled, intensive care at all hours. All thirty-five hospitals have intensive care units (see Table 6–9).

Many analysts believe that the high number of deaths from myocardial infarctions could be reduced by specialized coronary care units.[28] Twenty-six of the thirty-five Connecticut hospitals have separate coronary care units in addition to the aforementioned intensive care units.

Table 6-8.   Primary Support Services
Recommended Criteria for Emergency Departments
How Connecticut Hospitals Measure Up to Professional Standards

Primary Support Services	*The American College of Surgeons*	*The American Medical Association*	*Hospital Council Southern California*	*JCAH*	*Emergency Departments in Connecticut* #	*Emergency Departments in Connecticut* %
blood bank	X	X	X	X	35	100
blood bank in operation 24 hours a day	X	X	X		27	77
X-ray facilities in operation 24 hours a day	X	X	X	X	22	62
complete X-ray including angiography	X	X			34	97
portable X-ray available 24 hours a day					22	63
X-ray facilities located in the emergency department	X				6	17
laboratory facilities located in the emergency department	X				2	6

Table 6-9. Hospital Support Facilities
Recommended Criteria for Emergency Departments
How Connecticut Hospitals Measure Up to Professional Standards

	Recommended By:				Emergency Departments in Connecticut	
Hospital Support Facilities	*The American College of Surgeons*	*The American Medical Association*	*Hospital Council Southern California*	*JCAH*	#	%
intensive care unit	X	X	X		35	100
coronary care unit	X	X	X		26	74
operating room available 24 hours a day	X	X	X		16	45
postoperative recovery room 24 hours a day	X	X	X		25	71

Operating room facilities and postoperative recovery rooms must be available at all times if major trauma is to be managed effectively. Only 45 percent of Connecticut hospitals have their operating rooms staffed around-the-clock (see Table 6–9). This support service should be a major factor in categorization of EDs.

DISASTER PLANNING

An important dimension of emergency care is the ability to respond to mass casualties and major disasters. When a disaster occurs, whether it be a flood, fire, civil disorder, or industrial accident, the hospital becomes the focal point for the disposition and treatment of the injured. A sudden and massive influx of patients can overwhelm hospital facilities. The JCAH requires that each accredited hospital have a written plan for the care of mass casualties, and that the hospital perform two disaster drills each year. The AMA categorization guidelines require that all hospital emergency facilities must be prepared to expand its facilities when disaster strikes: "A mass casualty plan and the well-rehearsed capability to deliver emergency medical care for natural disasters or national emergencies shall be required. Ready access to supplemental space, equipment, supplies, and drugs is necessary."[29]

Although all hospitals have a disaster plan and a disaster planning committee, 20 percent performed no trial runs during 1970. Only 45 percent reported holding two or more disaster exercises. Indeed, 63 percent admitted that their present plan was inadequate.

We found that all thirty-five hospitals have supplemental power sources designed to give the emergency department 100 percent capability in the case of a power breakdown. Only 30 percent of the EDs maintain a designated stockpile of supplies to be used in disaster situations. Most Connecticut hospitals must improve their disaster preparedness if they are to fulfill their mission in the event of disaster.

SUMMARY OF FINDINGS

An examination of Connecticut hospital emergency departments reveals a large increase in patient visits from 1960 to 1974 (262 percent). All thirty-five emergency departments provide some form of medical coverage twenty-four hours a day and the majority have physician specialists on call around-the-clock. Most EDs maintain the recommended resuscitation equipment and "emergency trays" necessary for lifesaving therapy. However, some share equipment (defibrillators, electrocardiographs, and cardioscopes) with other hospital departments. While all EDs are guided by written policies and procedures, deficiencies were noted regarding the policies required by the Joint Commission on Accreditation of Hospitals. All thirty-five hospitals reported having a general intensive care unit and three-fourths have an additional coronary care unit functioning twenty-four hours a day.

Substantial emergency department construction and overhaul is in progress, indicating a responsiveness of the hospitals to meet increased utilization. Compared to information reported from most other states, Connecticut hospital emergency departments measure up rather well. They also measure up rather well when compared to other elements of EMS in Connecticut. The data collected in this chapter could serve as the basis for structural categorization of the state's emergency departments (see Chapter 11).

✳ *Chapter 7*

Emergency Department Physicians

INTRODUCTION AND OBJECTIVES

In 1966, an American Medical Association manual entitled *The Emergency Department: A Handbook for Medical Staff* presented two models of contractual agreements between hospitals and physicians for the purpose of staffing hospital emergency departments (EDs). The first model was based on an arrangement inaugurated in 1960 at Alexandria Hospital in Alexandria, Virginia.[1] The institution provided coverage with four full-time ED physicians, replacing the previous pattern of house officers and attending staff. The four practitioners were members of the hospital medical staff but were not allowed to have admitting privileges or an outside practice. They were to use their clinical discretion in making specialty referrals and a roster of specialists on "second-call" was maintained for this purpose. Each physician had the option of billing the patient directly or through the hospital, in which case the latter retained a 15 percent collection fee.

The second model was a partnership of attending staff physicians instituted in 1961 at Pontiac General Hospital in Pontiac, Michigan.[2] Twenty-three practitioners were included in the organization, and all retained some form of private practice. No participation eligibility distinction was made on the basis of specialty and the group's specialties included general practice, obstetrics, internal medicine, pediatrics, and general surgery. During the past decade, variations of the Alexandria and Pontiac plans as well as other models have emerged.

This chapter will focus on the physicians who staff the emergency departments of Connecticut's thirty-five acute general hospitals. It will present a profile of ED physicians, and will explore alternative direct-coverage arrangements, specialty physician backup, the trend toward hospital-based physician coverage, and deficiencies in current methods of training and continuing education for physicians in emergency care.

STAFFING PATTERNS

Connecticut's emergency departments utilize ten different staffing arrangements. The following five are uniform direct-coverage patterns in which the same mode of staffing is maintained at all times:

1. Salaried ED-based physicians working in an unincorporated group
2. Salaried ED-based physicians working in an incorporated group
3. Hospital-paid attending staff members
4. Nonhospital-paid attending staff members
5. Interns and residents.

One of these patterns is used at twenty-five of the thirty-five hospitals studied. The remaining ten institutions utilize five other modes of direct physician coverage, all of which are combinations of two or more of the above arrangements.

Twenty-three hospitals utilize salaried ED-based physicians to some extent. At fourteen EDs, they are the sole providers of coverage, while at nine hospitals they are employed in conjunction with members of the house staff or attending staff (see Table 7-1).

Attending staff physicians participate in ED coverage at fourteen institutions. At eight of these, they are the only mode of staffing. At six facilities, the participating attending staff members receive some form of remuneration from the hospital. Interns and residents provide coverage at nine institutions—exclusively at three and in combination with salaried ED-based physicians or members of the attending staff at six others (see Table 7-1).

The predominance of hospital-salaried, ED-based physician coverage is a relatively new phenomenon in Connecticut. To examine this development, we utilized an unpublished survey of ED physician staffing patterns conducted in 1966 by the Connecticut Academy of General Practice.[3] In 1966, the attending staff participated in ED coverage at twenty-five hospitals. Eight of these hospitals provided the physicians with some form of payment. Interns or residents

Table 7-1. Physician Staffing of Connecticut Hospital Emergency
Departments, 1971

Type of Arrangement	Number of Hospitals	Percent of Total
Nonincorporated group of salaried ED-based MDs	13	37
Incorporated group of salaried ED-based MDs	1	3
Rotation of hospital-paid attending staff	5	14
Salaried ED-based MDs with rotation of some hospital-paid attending staff	1	3
Salaried ED-based MDs with rotation of some nonhospital-paid attending staff	3	9
Rotation of some nonpaid members of the attending staff	3	9
Interns and/or residents	3	9
Interns and/or residents with salaried ED-based MDs	4	11
Interns and/or residents with rotation of some nonhospital-paid attending staff	1	3
Interns and/or residents with salaried ED-based MDs and rotation of some nonhospital-paid attending staff	1	3
Total	35	101

worked in the emergency departments of fourteen hospitals, at five
of which they were the sole providers of direct coverage. Of the
thirty-five institutions, only seven employed salaried ED-based physicians. This figure has tripled in five years (see Table 7-2).

The three hospitals that moved from rotation of nonhospital-paid
attending staff to complete coverage by salaried ED-based physicians
are relatively large (230 to 400 beds), and their ED utilization ranged
from approximately 13,000 to 40,000 visits for 1970. As one might
expect, the three facilities that changed from coverage by nonhospital-paid attending staff members to partial coverage with salaried ED-
based physicians are smaller, ranging from 120 beds to 200 beds.
Their ED utilization ranged from 9,000 to 19,000 visits for 1970.[a]

[a]Eight hospitals are planning to revise their staffing arrangements in the near
future. Of the three institutions that provide total coverage by salaried ED-based
MDs, two are planning to add new positions for "dual-coverage" arrangements,
and the third is contemplating consolidation of many part-time salaried slots
into several full-time positions. Another institution plans to replace part of its
nonhospital-paid attending staff with salaried ED-based physicians. A fifth hospital envisions expansion of partial coverage by salaried ED-based MDs to a com-

Table 7-2.   Selected Physician Staffing Patterns, 1966 and 1971

	1966		1971	
Type of Arrangement	Number of Hospitals	Percent	Number of Hospitals	Percent
Some attending staff members providing exclusive coverage	16	46	8	23
Some attending staff members involved in combination arrangement	9	26	6	17
Interns and/or residents providing exclusive coverage	5	14	3	9
Interns and/or residents involved in combination arrangement	9	26	6	17
Salaried ED-based MDs providing exclusive coverage	3	9	14	40
Salaried ED-based MDs involved in combination arrangement	4	11	9	26

The twenty-five hospitals that use one of the five single-coverage patterns were analyzed according to bed size and emergency department utilization. As expected, the small rural hospitals have maintained the rotation of nonhospital-paid attending staff members, while larger community hospitals have instituted a rotation with some hospital-paid members of the attending staff or with a group of salaried ED-based practitioners. Only the larger urban medical centers utilize interns and residents.

The pattern of coverage varies widely among the ten hospitals utilizing a combination staffing arrangement. At four institutions with interns or residents, the house staff covers the emergency service only during the day and under the supervision of members of the attending staff or salaried ED-based physicians, who in turn provide the remaining coverage. At two other institutions, interns or residents cover the emergency service at all times, but during the days and evenings they serve in conjunction with physicians on the attending staff or with salaried EMS practitioners.

Of the four hospitals utilizing a combination of attending staff and salaried ED-based physicians, two employ the latter to cover the emergency service on weekends and holidays; one of these two institutions also employs a full-time physician for the day shift during the week. The remaining two facilities take opposite approaches. One utilizes attending staff physicians on weekdays, with evening, night,

plete coverage arrangement with full-time practitioners. Two teaching hospitals plan to increase participation of the resident staff in the emergency department.

and weekend coverage provided by salaried ED-based MDs. The second employs a full-time, salaried ED-based physician for weekdays, with the rest of the coverage provided by the attending staff.

STAFFING LEVELS

All thirty-five hospitals have a first-call physician designated to cover the emergency department around-the-clock. Twenty-two hospitals have the equivalent of one physician staffing the emergency department for all shifts, and two others maintain constant physician manpower levels for every shift. One of the hospitals with constant physician manpower levels has the equivalent of three physicians covering medicine, surgery, and pediatrics; the other has six doctors covering the medical, surgical, pediatric, and psychiatric services. The remaining eleven hospitals employ different combinations of physicians to adapt the level of staffing to shift differentials in patient utilization.[b]

Another description of staffing levels can be made by defining the number of full-time physician equivalents (FTPEs). This approach yields a useful criterion for comparison and helps relate staffing level to patient utilization.

Table 7-3 illustrates the wide variation in utilization within each staffing level. The wide variation in visit-per-week utilization for the twenty-two hospitals with 4.2 physician manpower equivalents reflects in part the need to have at least one physician staffing the emergency department around-the-clock. However, four of the institutions at this minimum staffing level average more than 500 patient visits a week, implying some degree of understaffing compared to other hospitals.

Further variation in physician staffing/patient utilization ratios is revealed in Table 7-4, which demonstrates that this ratio varies eight-fold (0.22 MD man-hours/visit to 1.77 MD man-hours/visit) among those hospitals that require physician presence in the emergency department. Subsequent analysis shows that hospitals with small patient utilization rates have higher MD man-hour/visit ratios than those with higher utilization rates.[4] Although levels of staffing are related to utilization, an increase in the latter does not necessarily produce a commensurate increase in the former.

[b]One large metropolitan hospital utilizing a combination of interns and salaried ED-based MDs utilizes the following sub-shift coverage arrangements:

7 A.M.–10 A.M.: 1 MD	6 P.M.– 9 P.M.: 3 MDs
10 A.M.– 5 P.M.: 2 MDs	9 P.M.– 1 A.M.: 2 MDs
5 P.M.– 6 P.M.: 4 MDs	1 A.M.–7 A.M.: 1 MD

Table 7-3.   Distribution of Hospitals and Utilization Rates According to the Levels of Physician Staffing in the Emergency Department, 1970

Number of MD Man-Hours per Week	Number of Full-Time (40 hrs.) MD Equivalents	Number of Hospitals[a]	Average Number of Visits per Week	Range in Average Number of Visits per Week
168	4.2	22	319	59–760
176	4.4	2	572	411–774
184	4.6	1	402	—
192	4.8	1	741	—
208	5.2	1	758	—
224	5.6	2	507	373–641
280	7.0	1	386	—
376	9.4	1	740	—
504	12.6	1	365	—
728	18.2	1	778	—
784	19.6	1	1,102	—
1,008	25.2	1	1,525	—

[a]Includes three hospitals at the 4.2 FTPE level where the attending staff is on call to the emergency department.

Table 7–4 also shows that ED physicians spend an average of twenty minutes or less with each patient at seven of the hospitals. Because these statistics do not account for the day-night differential in utilization nor the extent of nonurgent treatment, a definitive judgment on the magnitude of any staffing inadequacy requires a significantly more detailed information base.

SPECIALTY BACKUP

Because of the unpredictability of ED visits, the most appropriate medical response will not always be within the clinical purview of the first-call physician. Thus the first-call MD must always have specialist backup. The Joint Commission on the Accreditation of Hospitals and the Committee on Trauma of the American College of Surgeons stress this point.[5] All thirty-five hospitals maintain policies and procedures to assure the availability of clinical specialty services to the emergency department on a second-call basis. (The services reported by Connecticut hospitals are presented in Table 7–5.)

Most hospitals (*n* = 25) report a "special-response" team within their institution. These teams are designed to give immediate treatment to cardiac patients, although other response capabilities were mentioned. They are comprised of physicians, nurses, and, in some instances, ancillary personnel for inhalation or intravenous therapy. Of the eight hospitals not having special-response teams, four are small community hospitals (under 150 beds) and three are intermediate-sized community hospitals (150–400 beds).

BACKGROUND, EDUCATION, AND TRAINING

To document the attitudes and practices of physicians engaged in emergency care, a study population based on the physician-hospital relationship was selected (see Chapter 2). The patterns of response among full-time (*n* = 51) and part-time (*n* = 58) ED physicians often varied, and in some cases the differences were significant.

The average age of the physicians in the study sample was forty-four years, although the diversity in ages was wide (see Table 7–6). The relatively low number of respondents in the thirty-one to thirty-five age range seems to indicate that many physicians, after completing specialty training, embark upon other careers before entering emergency care. Less than 11 percent of the group are over sixty-one. This finding contradicts a widely held impression that general practitioners often retire into hospital-based emergency care. The

Table 7-4.   Analysis of Hospitals According to Emergency Department Utilization Rates and Physician Manpower Staffing Characteristics, 1970

Hospital Number	Number of MD Man-Hours per Week	Number of Full-Time Equivalents	Number of Weekly Visits to the Emergency Department	MD Man-Hours per Visit	Weekly Visits per Full-Time MD Equivalent
1	168	4.2	760	0.22	180.1
2	176	4.4	734	0.24	166.7
3	192	4.8	741	0.26	154.3
4	208	5.2	758	0.27	145.8
5	168	4.2	577	0.29	137.3
6	168	4.2	549	0.31	130.7
7	168	4.2	520	0.32	123.8
8	224	5.6	641	0.35	114.5
9	168	4.2	474	0.35	112.8
10	168	4.2	464	0.36	110.5
11	168	4.2	457	0.37	108.7
12	376	9.4	940	0.40	100.0
13	168	4.2	417	0.40	99.4
14	176	4.4	411	0.43	93.4
15	168	4.2	380	0.44	90.4

16	168	4.2	378	0.45	89.9
17	168	4.2	364	0.46	86.8
18	184	4.6	402	0.46	86.6
19	168	4.2	311	0.54	74.0
20	168	4.2	308	0.55	73.3
21	224	5.6	373	0.60	66.5
22	168	4.2	263	0.64	62.7
23	1008	25.2	1525	0.66	60.5
24	784	19.6	1102	0.71	56.2
25	280	7.0	386	0.72	55.2
26	728	18.2	778	0.94	42.7
27	168	4.2	175	0.96	41.7
28	504	12.6	365	1.38	28.9
29	168	4.2	118	1.42	28.1
30	168	4.2	105	1.60	25.0
31	168	4.2	97	1.74	23.0
32	168	4.2	95	1.77	22.6
33[a]	168	4.2	69	2.44[a]	16.3
34[a]	168	4.2	68	2.46[a]	16.3
35	168	4.2	59	2.86[a]	14.0

[a]Physician on call to emergency department.

Table 7-5. Analysis of Hospitals According to the Clinical Specialties on Second Call to the Emergency Department, 1970

Clinical Specialty Available on Second Call	Number of Hospitals Providing Specialty	Percent of Hospitals Providing Specialty
General Surgery	35	100
Internal Medicine	35	100
OBS/GYN	35	100
Pediatrics	34	97
Ophthalmology	34	97
Orthopedic Surgery	33	94
Anesthesiology	33	94
Radiology	33	94
ENT	32	91
Pathology	32	91
Cardiology	31	89
Psychiatry	31	89
Neurosurgery	25	71
Plastic Surgery	25	71
Neurology	21	60

part-time practitioners were, in general, considerably younger than their full-time counterparts (see Table 7-7). This difference may be attributable to several factors. First, the part-time category includes physicians who have not yet entered a formal practice of their own. Some are residents at other hospitals; others are medical officers performing their active duty obligation at a nearby military institution. The willingness of these physicians to participate in ED coverage at an earlier age may also reflect the financial incentives offered by the institution.

The inverse tends to characterize the full-time group. As documented later, most full-time ED physicians have selected emergency care subsequent to a substantial involvement in private practice. The majority of the full-time group are between the ages of forty-one and

Table 7-6. Distribution of ED Physicians According to Age

Age Range	Number of MDs	Percent of MDs
30 and under	13	12
31–35	6	6
36–40	16	15
41–45	14	13
46–50	15	14
51–55	20	18
56–60	13	12
61–65	8	7
66–70	3	3
Total	108	100

Table 7-7. EMS Physician Age Range Comparisons According to the Extent of Involvement in the Emergency Department

Age Range	Number of Full-Time MDs	Percent of Full-Time MDs	Number of Part-Time MDs	Percent of Part-Time MDs
30 and under	2	4	11	19
31–35	2	4	4	7
36–40	3	6	13	22
41–45	8	16	6	10
46–50	10	20	5	9
51–55	8	16	12	21
56–60	9	18	4	7
61–65	6	12	2	3
66–70	2	4	1	2
Total	50	100	58	100

Note: $x^2 = 19.31$, $p < 0.05$ with 8 degrees of freedom.

fifty-five. These physicians did not retire to emergency service work but entered EMS practice in midcareer.

Most ED physicians ($n = 88$) served a one-year internship; the other fourteen served internships of two or three years. Many of the extended internships were multiple clinical rotations or surgical programs that existed prior to 1950. Although there was a degree of specialization at that level, most internships were mixed clinical programs. Twenty-eight physicians terminated their formal training after internship. Of these, twenty-five completed a mixed internship program, and the remaining three served either a straight medical or surgical program. Of the eighty ED physicians who received residency training, few were residents for longer than three years (see Table 7-8).

Sixty-six physicians provided information on their clinical specialty training, which in most cases was in medicine or surgery.

Table 7-8. Distribution of ED Physicians by Length of Residency Training

Number of Years	Number of MDs	Percent of Total
1	29	38
2	20	26
3	16	21
4	8	10
5	3	4
7	1[a]	1
Total	77	100

[a]The one physician with seven years of residency training was involved in several programs.

Table 7-9.   Distribution of ED Physicians by Specialty of Residency Training

Specialty	Number of MDs	Percent of Total
Surgery	20	30
Medicine	17	36
Surgery and other specialty	7	11
Medicine and other specialty	7	11
Pediatrics	5	8
Mixed	4	6
General practice	3	4
Other	3	4
Total	66	98

Eighty-nine physicians (82 percent) received formal training in an emergency department during internship or residency. The emergency department rotation averaged 3.3 months in length. Of the sixteen physicians who did not have formal ED training, ten are now full-time and six are part-time ED physicians.

Thirty-three ED physicians received some postgraduate training in emergency care. As illustrated in Table 7-10, the substantial majority of these doctors are in full-time ED practice. But nearly 45 percent of the full-time ED physicians have never participated in a postgraduate course in emergency medical treatment.

Twenty-two respondents (20 percent) were board certified. Only two of the full-time physicians were board certified. In contrast, twenty of fifty-seven part-time ED physicians were board certified ($p < 0.001$). Specialty certification of the part-time physicians included surgery ($n = 5$), family practice ($n = 5$), pediatrics ($n = 4$), and internal medicine ($n = 3$).

Table 7-10.   Analysis of EMS Physicians by Postgraduate Emergency-Care Training

Response	Number of Full-Time MDs	Percent of Full-Time MDs	Number of Part-Time MDs	Percent of Part-Time MDs
Have attended programs	27	55	6	11
Have not attended programs	22	45	50	89

Note: x^2 = 23.89, $p < 0.001$ with 1 degree of freedom.

Table 7-11. Previous Professional Capacity of the Full-Time ED Physicians

Professional Capacity	Number of MDs	Percent of Total
Private practice		
General practice	23	46
Internal medicine	8	16
Surgery	6	12
Neurology	1	2
Residency	5	10
Other hospital-based		
practice	2	4
School MDs	2	4
Others	3	6
Total	50	100

To identify characteristics of professional mobility, the full-time physicians were requested to define their medical capacity prior to entering emergency care (see Table 7-11). The greatest shift came from private general practice. Four of the five physicians who had just completed their residency training reported that they planned to stay in emergency medical work.

Prior to assuming their current position, more than half (57 percent) of the full-time physicians practiced within the immediate vicinity, and another 23 percent came from other communities within the state. Thus the largest source of full-time ED physician supply in Connecticut is the pool of general practitioners in the community served by the hospital.

Most part-time ED physicians are engaged in some concurrent form of private practice, though here the percentage of general practitioners is comparatively smaller (see Table 7-12). These statistics

Table 7-12. Concurrent Professional Capacity of the Part-Time ED Physicians

Professional Capacity	Number of MDs	Percent of Total
Private practice		
General practice	12	21
Internal medicine	6	10
Surgery	12	21
OBS/GYN	1	2
Pediatrics	4	7
Military MD	11	19
Moonlighting residents	3	5
Industrial medicine	3	5
Institutional medicine	3	5
Research	3	5
Total	58	100

may understate the role of "moonlighting" residents. Some hospitals discourage their house staff from moonlighting. Furthermore, one institution that employed a substantial number of moonlighting residents from a nearby medical center declined to participate in this part of the study in order to maintain the confidentiality of their working arrangements.

MOTIVATIONS FOR EMERGENCY MEDICAL PRACTICE

What do physicians see as the advantages of moving into full-time salaried ED positions? The potential incentives for the practice of emergency medicine are shown by order of importance in Table 7-13. A weighted numerical value was tabulated to facilitate aggregate comparisons.[c] According to the number of ranked responses and the corresponding weighted values, the primary reason for choosing emergency work was financial, followed by the predictability of hours on duty and a preference for providing acute medical care.

The full-time and part-time practitioners gave significantly different responses. The predictability of working hours was weighted most heavily among the full-time group which squares with the heavy time demands on many general practitioners (see Table 7-14). The part-time group weighted income advantages most heavily, as might be expected of younger physicians engaged principally in some other form of medical practice (see Table 7-15).

Another assessment of physician preference for ED work was obtained by exploring their career plans. Seventy-seven of the 101 MDs responding plan to stay in emergency medical practice. Forty-six of forty-nine full-time respondents expect to remain in ED work, while only thirty-one of fifty-two part-time physicians plan to do so ($p < 0.001$).

HOSPITAL-PHYSICIAN RELATIONSHIPS

Several elements of the hospital-physician relationship were explored, such as the time devoted to emergency department coverage,

---

[c]In order to arrive at this number, five points were assigned to each reason when it was listed as most important, four points when listed as second most important, and so on, with one point assigned for each reason that was ranked fifth or below. These subtotals were then summed. In those few instances where a physician checked only two reasons, both were considered most important. It should be emphasized that these values are meaningful only as a comparative index to the other scores.

Table 7-13. Comparison of Motivational Factors Influencing ED Physician Practice

Reasons for Becoming Involved in Emergency Department Practice	Number of Times Reason Was Given as:						Weighted Value of Reason
	Most Important	2nd in Importance	3rd in Importance	4th in Importance	5th in Importance	6th in Importance	
Preference for providing acute medical care	19	24	16	4	2	—	249
Preference for not having to provide long-term care	3	12	12	15	7	1	137
Facilitating patient contacts upon starting practice	2	3	2	1	12	7	49
Predictability of hours on duty	31	20	12	5	2	—	283
Financial and income advantages	35	16	12	12	2	—	301
Other	23	11	5	2	1	—	179

Table 7-14. Comparison of Motivational Factors Influencing Full-Time ED Physician Practice

Reasons for Becoming Involved in Emergency Department Practice	Number of Times Reason Was Given as:						Weighted Value of Reason
	Most Important	2nd in Importance	3rd in Importance	4th in Importance	5th in Importance	6th in Importance	
Preference for providing acute medical care	10	16	9	—	1	—	142
Preference for not having to provide long-term care	2	9	8	7	1	1	86
Facilitating patient contacts upon starting practice	—	1	—	—	5	3	12
Predictability of hours on duty	28	10	6	1	—	—	200
Financial and income advantages	3	7	5	9	2	—	78
Other	10	2	4	2	1	—	75

Table 7-15. Comparison of Motivational Factors Influencing Part-Time ED Physician Practice

Reasons for Becoming Involved in Emergency Department Practice	Number of Times Reason Was Given as:						Weighted Value of Reason
	Most Important	2nd in Importance	3rd in Importance	4th in Importance	5th in Importance	6th in Importance	
Preference for providing acute medical care	9	8	7	4	1	—	107
Preference for not having to provide long-term care	1	3	4	8	6	—	151
Facilitating patient contacts upon starting practice	2	2	2	1	7	4	37
Predictability of hours on duty	3	10	6	4	2	—	83
Financial and income advantages	32	9	7	3	—	—	223
Other[a]	13	9	1	—	—	—	104

[a]The reason most frequently given in the "Other" category cited the need for emergency care in the community and the participation of the physicians in fulfilling that need.

staff affiliations, other professional responsibilities within the institution, and hospital-physician financial arrangements. The full-time ED physician works an average of 39.9 hours per week. Nearly half of these physicians (n = 25) work a 40-hour week, but the range varies from 26 to 57 hours per week.[d] Part-time physicians devote an average of 57 hours per *month* to the coverage of the emergency department, although the range varies considerably from less than 20 hours to 140 hours per month.

More full-time physicians (72 percent) are accorded active staff privileges than their part-time counterparts (55 percent). This may be attributable to the implied expression of prolonged commitment inherent in a full-time position and the absence of that commitment in many part-time arrangements.[e]

As a rule, Connecticut physicians do not admit patients to their own hospital service when covering the emergency department. When patients require hospital admission, they are typically referred to a private physician or to the MD responsible for the respective clinical service. Provided that the emergency department MD and the physician of referral agree about the need for admission, the question of admitting privileges for the former becomes moot. However, if there were frequent discord over the need for admission, admitting privileges by the emergency department physician could become a central issue.

To explore this point, full-time physicians were asked if they possessed admitting privileges and if they deemed these privileges important to their ED practice. Of forty-nine respondents, only ten have admitting privileges, eight of whom stipulated that these privileges were important. The assurance that seriously ill patients would be admitted promptly was the reason most frequently mentioned.

The inhospital responsibilities of ED physicians were also explored. Because a large portion of the part-time group were paid attending staff members with responsibilities commensurate with full membership on the active staff, they were not questioned on this point. Only the additional responsibilities of full-time MDs were considered. Of the fifty-one physicians who work full time, thirty-one reported hospital responsibilities beyond the emergency department. Almost half mentioned their participation on assorted medical staff

[d]Several physicians who work less than thirty-five hours a week were included in this category if their work in the emergency service constitutes their only professional activity.

[e]The divergence of active staff appointments between the two groups would have been more pronounced if the paid attending staff members were excluded from the part-time physician sample.

committees. Another eight listed coverage of the employee health service, and six mentioned the responsibility of covering inhospital emergencies either as a formal member of a cardiac-arrest team or simply when other physicians were not readily available. Additional duties included teaching house staff, teaching nursing personnel, and general clinic coverage.

A variety of methods of payment for ED physicians emerged with salary arrangements most common. In some cases, the physician receives a percentage of charges for patient services billed by the hospital, with the institution usually guaranteeing a minimum income. A majority of both full-time and part-time practitioners receive a straight salary from the hospital, but a much higher proportion of part-time practitioners are paid according to a percentage of patient charges. A high proportion of the paid attending staff members are remunerated under this modified fee-for-service mechanism.

Three major issues were examined regarding the professional relationship between ED physicians and other members of the attending staff. First, ED physicians were asked to estimate utilization of specialty backup services in proportion to their own patient loads. These data reflect the extent of clinical interaction and the perceived degree of diagnostic and therapeutic self-sufficiency attributable to the emergency department MD. Secondly, because ED physicians often assume the surrogate role of a "community" physician, this role was assessed through the nonemergency utilization of the emergency department by private patients of other physicians. The third issue was the designation of inpatient medical responsibility for patients admitted through the ED.

Physicians were requested to indicate, with respect to their total patient load, the percentage of cases in which they obtained either a specialty consultation, a specialty referral (including hospital admission), or a direct patient transfer to another medical facility. Approximately two-thirds of 104 physician respondents report that they attend exclusively more than 90 percent of the patients that they see in the ED. When the range of frequencies was analyzed according to full- and part-time relationships, no obvious differences appeared.

The specialties routinely utilized were listed by 102 physicians. Surgery was mentioned by 78 percent and orthopedics by 66 percent. Other frequently reported specialty consultations included medicine (49 percent), pediatrics (30 percent), ophthalmology (20 percent), psychiatry (19 percent), ENT (19 percent), and Obs/Gyn (18 percent).

Documentation of the nonurgent, private patient utilization was not possible. But in order to demonstrate the association between such utilization and the full-time presence of a physician in the ED, the function of the physician in the treatment of these nonurgent cases was examined. ED physicians estimated that they treat exclusively 58 percent of cases, that they treat 25 percent of patients subsequent to referral by a private physician, and that 17 percent of patients are treated exclusively by the private physician. Even though these statistics are only the averages of estimates, they give at least a rough impression of the utilization of the ED physician by the patients of other practitioners.

The use of the ED physician to provide nonurgent episodic medical care for the private patients of other physicians probably results from several factors. First, when patients decide to seek medical treatment for a nonurgent problem, they are often able to be seen much more quickly in the ED than in their own doctor's office. Second, when the private physician is not readily available, especially at night, his office often refers patients to the emergency department. Third, when presented with a choice of receiving office-type care from two sources in the community, the private patient often selects the hospital if he believes that his insurance will then cover the service.

Although policies outlining medical responsibilities are formulated by the medical staff at each hospital, the full-time presence of an in-hospital ED physician may have an effect on the responsibilities normally assumed by the attending staff. Of particular interest was the extent of responsibility for patients admitted to the hospital through the ED. Although the physician of referral theoretically assumes responsibility upon admission of the patient, in actual practice if this physician is unable to attend to the patient immediately the responsibility may be maintained by the ED physician. ED physicians were asked to designate whom they believed to be the responsible physician for patients admitted through the emergency department prior to the arrival of the physician of referral. Table 7–16 indicates the diversity of their views.

Of the qualified responses that favored the admitting physician, several alluded to the shift of responsibility to the physician of referral as soon as the patient left the emergency department. Of the two qualified responses that favored the ED physician, one stipulated that the physician "on service" be unavailable, and the other stated that the responsibility of the ED physician should end one hour after the patient was admitted. Most of the responses in the "Other" category maintained that the MD on service was responsible.

Table 7-16. Distribution of ED Physicians According to the Designation of Medical Responsibility for Patients Admitted through the Emergency Department

Designation of Responsible Physician	*Number of MDs*	*Percent of MDs*
Emergency service MD	26	27
Admitting MD	25	26
House staff	14	14
Emergency service MD and house staff	11	11
Admitting physician (response qualified)	9	9
Emergency service MD (response qualified)	2	2
Other combinations	10	10
Total	97	99

When essentially the same question was posed to the hospitals, nearly two out of three placed the responsibility with the ED physician, while the remainder assigned the responsibility to the admitting MD.

EDUCATION IN EMERGENCY CARE

ED physicians were questioned about the need for a program of emergency care education in Connecticut. Practitioners were asked to select those topics that they considered most needed for their continuing education and what they considered to be the optimal educational background for EMS physicians.

The physicians report they spend an average of seventeen hours per month on various self-educational activities about two-thirds of which are devoted to reading (see Table 7-17).[6]

Table 7-17. Average Hours per Month Devoted to Self-Education in Emergency Care by ED Physicians

Method of Self-Education	*Average Hours per Month*
Conferences and group discussions	2.4
Reading	11.2
Formal training	0.3
Patient case review	1.0
Audiovisual methods	0.5
Other	1.4
Total	16.8

Less than half (n = 52) of the ED physicians believe their current educational resources were sufficient to keep up with the latest developments in emergency medical practice. Over 90 percent favor attending postgraduate courses in emergency care if such courses could be made conveniently available. Physicians were asked to select those areas they judged most important from a list of fifteen possible topics. Ranked according to the frequency of selection, the seven most important topics are:

1. Cardiopulmonary resuscitation (including defibrillation and intubation)
2. Management of pediatric emergencies
3. Management of major trauma
4. Treatment of cardiac arrhythmias and EKG reading
5. Management of the comatose patient (including laboratory interpretations)
6. Management of drug abuse and alcoholism
7. Advances in toxicology and pharmacology.

The prime importance attached to cardiac resuscitation reflects not only the high incidence of cardiac cases seen in emergency departments but also the recognized association between proper therapeutic technique and optimal therapeutic outcome in these situations. The relatively high importance of the management of pediatric emergencies may be indicative of the few physicians (n = 5) with formal training in pediatrics. With the exception of major trauma management, surgical procedures received comparatively lower ratings, possibly reflecting the prevalence of physicians with surgical residency training.

A variety of responses were received on the question of preferred professional backgrounds for physicians involved in emergency care. Thirty-six percent of ED physicians believe that general practice provides the best background, 20 percent list special residencies in emergency care, and 5 percent prefer general surgery. The remaining 39 percent suggest combinations involving specialty residencies, general surgery, and general practice.

The question of board certification is an issue of growing concern for ED practitioners. Regarding the desirability of establishing board certification in emergency medical practice, forty-eight are in favor and forty-eight are opposed. Not surprisingly, there are significant differences between the full-time and part-time practitioners. The strength of support for board certification rests with the full-time physicians, who voted two to one in favor. Part-time physicians are opposed by a three to two margin. Details of certification preferences were quite diverse. The majority favor combinations of special residencies, specified years of experience, and demonstrated ability through board examinations.

SUMMARY OF FINDINGS

One of the most striking findings of our study of ED physician manpower is its organizational diversity. Ten different staffing patterns exist, and not one is common to a majority of the hospitals. Less than 50 percent of the institutions designate one ED physician as specifically in charge of the emergency department. There are also a variety of clinical specialists serving in second-call capacities. More than half of Connecticut institutions plan to modify their physician coverage patterns within the near future.

Another significant variation in physician manpower relates to staffing levels. Although the level of staffing appears dependent upon patient use in individual hospital emergency departments, variations in MD manpower-per-visit statistics indicate that the level of staffing is not consistent with utilization. The variance reflects in part the minimum requirement of having at least one physician on call at all times, regardless of low utilization, in addition to the specialty service, as well as dual-coverage arrangements involving the participation of the house staff. The absence of staffing guidelines for determining the adequacy of the levels of physician coverage is clear.

The rapid rise in ED utilization has stimulated changes in staffing arrangements over the last five years. Hospitals have taken steps to provide patients direct access to the physician covering the emergency department. A strong indicator of these steps is the move to employ full-time salaried physicians in the ED. In 1966, twelve institutions relied exclusively on the voluntary participation of the attending staff, while in 1971 only three hospitals did. Not surprisingly, those three facilities have the lowest patient-utilization rates of all thirty-five hospitals. Most full-time ED physicians move into this work from private practice in midcareer and from the immediate vicinity of the hospital. Their principal reason for making the change is predictability of working hours. Part-time ED physicians cite income advantages as their principal attraction. Nearly all full-time ED physicians expect to remain in ED work.

The need for continuing education is clear. Most of the practitioners believe that their present educational resources are insufficient to keep them aware of the latest developments in emergency care, and only one-third attended formal continuing-education programs.

Nine out of ten physicians expressed an interest in attending a post-graduate program in emergency care, yet less than a quarter of the institutions offered any continuing-education programs for physicians. Training in cardiopulmonary resuscitation and in the management of pediatric emergencies were listed as topics of greatest interest.

Emergency Department Nurses and Other ED Personnel

INTRODUCTION AND OBJECTIVES

The increased demands on hospital emergency department and their physician manpower extend to nurses and other health personnel in the ED. Here, too, a significant part of any improvement in emergency care depends upon appropriate training and upgrading of skills. This chapter will examine the role of registered nurses (RNs), licensed practical nurses (LPNs), aides/orderlies (A/Os), and "other EMS personnel" employed in Connecticut's thirty-five hospital emergency departments.

The chapter's objectives are to obtain a basic profile of nurses and other health personnel who work in Connecticut hospital EDs, to explore the receptivity of these personnel and their supervising physicians to expanded clinical roles, and to review current staffing patterns using a regression formula. Quantitative descriptors (age, sex, race, employment status, wages, etc.) and qualitative descriptors (a person's view of his own capabilities and performance) are employed (see Chapter 2). In discussing current staffing patterns, we develop ratios that contrast scheduled man-hours to visits as well as ratios indicating scheduled man-hours by personnel category.

A PROFILE OF ED NURSES AND OTHER ED PERSONNEL

Registered nurses constitute the largest personnel group we studied, with 359 questionnaires distributed and 256 (71 percent) returned. Of the RNs who responded, 167 (64 percent) were full-time and 89 (35 percent) were part-time employees. Questionnaires were distributed to fifty-two licensed practical nurses and thirty (58 percent) completed questionnaires were returned. Of these, twenty-six (87 percent) were from full-time and four (13 percent) from part-time personnel.

There were ninety-three questionnaires distributed to the aide/orderly group (A/Os), of which fifty-nine (63 percent) were completed. Of the fifty-nine completed questionnaires, forty-eight (81 percent) were from full-time and eleven (19 percent) from part-time A/Os. The "other EMS personnel" category was the smallest and most diverse. Fifteen questionnaires were distributed and ten (67 percent) were returned—six for full-time and four for part-time employees. Six of the ten respondents carried the job title of "surgical technician," two were "EKG technicians," and one was a "student nurse."

Demographic Characteristics

As expected, most RNs employed in emergency departments are women; only one questionnaire was returned by a male nurse. Almost half of the study group is under thirty and only three of the respondents (1 percent) are nonwhite. Most LPNs are female (97 percent) and white (90 percent) but vary widely in age.

The aides/orderlies constitute two distinct groups by age. The median age of the full-time A/Os is thirty-one, while median age of the part-time A/Os is twenty-one. Most part-time A/Os are male (73 percent), all are white, and many are college students on summer jobs. The full-time A/Os are evenly divided between men and women and one-fourth are nonwhite. The "other EMS personnel" group has a median age of twenty-six, two-thirds are male, and all are white.

Economic Characteristics

Full-time RNs receive a median hourly wage of $4.50 in contrast to part-time RNs whose hourly median is $4.34. The payment of shift differentials, usually expressed as a percentage of the base hourly rate, is standard practice throughout the state for many occupations. The median shift differentials for RNs working evenings and nights are $0.41 and $0.40 per hour, respectively. The payment of any wage differential for emergency department work (compared to other hospital work) is limited for all occupations, and only 4 percent of the RNs reported such a differential. The modal response for emergency department differentials is $0.05 per hour (three of seven responses).

The median hourly rate for LPNs is $3.40, with little variation between part-time and full-time employees. Evening and night shift differentials are $0.34 per hour for evenings and $0.35 for nights. Only five (17 percent) of the LPNs receive a pay differential for ED work. The modal response for ED differentials is $0.05 per hour (three responses).

Part-time aides/orderlies are paid $2.42 per hour, while full-time A/Os receive $2.74 per hour. Only two receive salary differentials for ED work. The median hourly wage for "other EMS personnel" is $2.68.

Education, Training, and Experience

Ninety-two percent of the registered nurses staffing Connecticut emergency departments are graduates of diploma schools of nursing. Six percent have baccalaureate degrees, and the remainder have master's (0.5 percent) or associate degrees (1 percent). Twenty percent were trained in Connecticut.

Most RNs begin their nursing careers in areas other than emergency medical service and then move to the ED. Only 46 percent of RNs received special training in emergency care. The types of training received are shown in Table 8–1, which reveals an emphasis on cardiopulmonary training. Fewer part-time RNs receive EMS training than full-time RNs (54 percent vs. 34 percent). Twelve percent of RNs perform special duties in areas of the hospital other than the ED. Of these, taking EKGs and giving IV therapy are most common.

Table 8–1. EMS Training for RNs in Connecticut Emergency Departments

Type of Training	Number of RNs
Cardiopulmonary resuscitation and/or coronary care	43
Requirement for degree[a]	31
On-the-job	19
Vehicle trauma	19
American College of Surgeons postgraduate	8
Other	16
Place of Training	
Hospital based	117
Nonhospital based	18
Not specified	1

[a]The "requirement for degree" category was not well defined by the respondents and included scheduled rotations through the ED as well as classes that were part of the standard curriculum for RNs.

Approximately 90 percent of LPNs are graduates of twelve-month training programs, while 10 percent have completed eighteen-month programs. Eighty-four percent are high school graduates and 13 percent have had some college education. Only ten (36 percent) of the LPNs received specific training in the care of acutely ill or injured patients.

The majority of the aides/orderlies are high school graduates only. In preparation for work in the medical field, 43 percent of the A/Os had formal, documented, on-the-job training, while 57 percent received informal on-the-job training. Two-thirds received general patient care or nurse's aide training. Eighty-four percent received the equivalent of four weeks or less of training and only 31 percent were trained in handling seriously ill or injured patients.

All of the "other EMS personnel" group completed high school, three had some college education, and one completed a vocational school course. One-third received formal on-the-job medical training, seven had military medical training, and five (50 percent) received emergency medical training. Three perform job specialties in other areas of the hospital—two doing EKGs and one doing cast work.

Job Motivation

Ninety-four percent of the registered nurses prefer emergency medical care work to work in other areas of the hospital. The most desirable qualities of ED work listed were opportunities for change, excitement, and challenge; the least desirable were routine work with nonemergent patients and dissatisfaction caused by lack of patient follow-up or staffing problems. Ninety-six percent were willing to take additional training while on duty at the hospital's expense, and 48 percent would take training offered outside the hospital at their own expense.

The licensed practical nurses responded similarly with 90 percent preferring EMS work to other types of work available for LPNs in hospitals. Eighty-three percent choose to work in the ED and the LPNs also described much the same qualities as "most desirable" and "least desirable" as RNs did. A high percentage (96 percent) responded favorably to taking additional training programs, but this varied from 52 percent to 96 percent, depending on whether or not personal expense would be incurred. A/Os and other EMS personnel responded similarly. All the ED personnel seem to be attracted to emergency department work by its variety, challenge, and learning opportunities.

PROFILE OF EXISTING AND
PREFERRED JOB FUNCTIONS

Recognizing the trends in nursing and other health occupations toward expanded roles, we attempted to obtain a picture of job functions and preferences for each personnel category in the hospital emergency department.[1] This section provides some insight into the receptivity of each personnel group toward expanded job roles.

Two types of task responses were sought from each personnel group. One was the open-ended, qualitative question asking for a "yes" or "no" judgment followed by a list of relevant tasks for all positive responses. The other presented a list of forty-three types of medical-surgical tasks and solicited eight possible responses for each. (See Chapter 2 for the details of the methodology employed.)

Table 8-2 shows the overall receptivity of each personnel group to an enlarged job role. In each category, more than half the respondents felt capable of performing tasks more difficult or responsible than those they routinely performed. LPNs gave the lowest positive response of the four categories; RNs and other EMS personnel registered the highest. Table 8-3 lists the most commonly cited of these "more responsible/difficult" tasks. These examples are similar for each group and certain tasks (i.e., suturing, suture removals, and dressings) appear in all groups. But there is a distinct difference in the array of the tasks listed by RNs compared to the others.

Table 8-4 lists tasks that the RNs now perform but believe could be handled by persons with less education or training. Except for changing dressings and casts, none of these tasks appears in Table 8-3 as "more responsible tasks" desired by LPNs or the A/O group. Clearly, there are tasks associated with emergency medical care that no one *wants* to perform but that must be performed at all levels at one time or another.

Table 8-2.   Responses of Nonphysician Personnel in Connecticut Emergency Departments to the Question "Are You Now Capable of Performing More Responsible/Difficult Tasks Than You Are Routinely Given?"

	Yes		*No*	
Profession	*Number*	*Percent*	*Number*	*Percent*
RNs (*n*=253)	210	83	43	17
LPNs (*n*=28)	17	61	11	39
A/Os (*n*=55)	41	74	14	26
Other EMS (*n*=7) Personnel	6	84	1	14

Table 8-3.   Examples of More Responsible/Difficult Tasks That
Nonphysician Personnel in Connecticut Emergency Departments Believe
They Can Now Perform

RN Tasks (54 listed)	Number of Affirmative Responses
Start IV fluids	106
Suture minor lacerations	78
Remove sutures	57
Order X-rays and/or blood work	53
Pass nasogastric tubes	37
Perform EKGs	36
Draw blood	35
Change dressings and/or casts	32
Other (19 separate tasks listed)	113
LPN Tasks (28 listed)	
Give medication	6
Suture minor lacerations	4
Remove sutures	3
Give injections	2
Change dressings and/or casts	2
Other	7
Not specified	4
A/O Tasks (71 listed)	
Change dressings and/or casts	14
Prepare IVs	10
Suture minor lacerations	9
Remove sutures	9
Perform catheterizations	6
Give injections	5
Administer oxygen and medications	4
Perform advanced first-aid techniques	3
Perform EKGs	3
Not specified	17
Other EMS Personnel Tasks (12 listed)	
Suture minor lacerations	4
Remove sutures	3
Give injections	2
Other	3

TASK ASSESSMENT BY PHYSICIANS AND NURSES

To explore the level of physician receptivity to role expansion by
RNs, we presented the basic task list to ED physicians and compared
their opinions with those of the nurses.[2] Selected tasks are presented

in five groups: (1) those that are performed by all or nearly all ED categories; (2) those that physicians feel only they should perform; (3) those that physicians or nurses only should perform; (4) those about which there is disagreement; and (5) those that lend themselves to further interpretation in each individual case. (See Chapter 2 for the methodology employed.)

In order for a task to be assigned to someone other than a physician, there had to be a high percentage of responses from physicians indicating willingness to delegate the task as well as a high percentage of responses from nonphysicians indicating willingness to perform it. Tasks were placed in the "disagreement group" (#4) if physicians would not delegate them despite nonphysician willingness to perform them, or if physicians would delegate them but nonphysicians felt them to be above their professional capabilities.

The following tasks are performed by all ED personnel categories:

- Apply tape or ace bandage to ankle, wrist, knee, or chest
- Apply a sling
- Apply splints to possible or untreated fractures of extremities
- Apply finger or hand splint
- Apply cervical collar
- Stop minor bleeding
- Clean wounds, cuts, abrasions
- Take and record vital signs
- Insert oropharyngeal airway (not performed by A/O)
- Perform electrocardiograms (with training).

These constitute a significant portion of the routine tasks performed in the emergency department. The following are tasks that physicians believe only they should perform:

Table 8-4. Examples of Responses by RNs in Connecticut Emergency Departments to Tasks That They Believe Could Be Performed by Persons with Less Education or Training

Tasks (534 listed)	*Number of Positive Responses*
Do paper work	112
Upkeep of treatment areas	78
Take temperature/pulse/respiration	62
Transport patients	45
Clean and wrap equipment sets	42
Housekeeping	33
Assist with minor suturing procedures	26
Do simple dressings and cast applications	22
Take blood pressures	18
Other	96

- Remove foreign body from external ear
- Remove foreign body from nares (nose)
- Remove foreign body from eye
- Control anterior nasal hemorrhage
- Suture superficial laceration
- Incise and drain small superficial abcess
- Insert packing into incision, wound, or cavity
- Reduce simple fracture
- Perform casting procedures
- Debride superficial wound or burn (some disagreement here)
- Check incisions, wounds, or burns for progress in healing
- Perform emergency tracheostomy
- Administer local anesthetics prior to suturing
- Perform history and physical examination
- Order laboratory tests (some disagreement here)
- Complete "return to work" permits
- Perform endotracheal intubation (some disagreement here).

Some of these tasks fall within the disagreement group and will be mentioned below. Many of the above tasks that have been customarily performed by the physician vary substantially in degree of responsibility or skill required.

The following tasks are generally recognized by physicians and nurses as appropriate for RNs to perform:

- Defibrillate cardiac patients as required
- Gastric lavage (some disagreement here)
- Clean ears of impacted wax (some disagreement here)
- Remove sutures
- Start an IV.

These tasks represent a diverse combination of responses. Basically, the physicians indicated a willingness to delegate the task to RNs, and the RN either had already performed the task or was willing to if given the proper training.

There is some disagreement between physician and nurse about the following tasks:

- Remove foreign body from external ear
- Remove foreign body from nares (nose)
- Suture superficial laceration
- Incise and drain small superficial abcess
- Insert packing into incision, wound, or cavity.

The disagreement cuts both ways, with either the physician un-willing to delegate or the RNs not eager to accept responsibility. The physicians were in large part (although not unanimously) willing to delegate removal of foreign bodies, but the RNs were undecided about it, with almost equal numbers willing and unwilling to accept the task. The disagreement was greater concerning suturing and in-cision and drainage of abcess and packing wounds. A large number of nurses were willing to undertake these tasks, but the physicians were not prepared to delegate them.

Several tasks lend themselves to interesting interpretations. The tasks involving cast work are felt by all categories to belong at the physician level. Starting an IV has a high degree of acceptance as an RN function, but relatively few RNs perform the task at present, and many feel a need for training in this function. Also, a large number of non-RNs are willing to accept this task, which lends credence to the current trend of training other personnel to administer intra-venous fluids.

Our exploration of expanded job functions for nurses and other ED personnel reveals a willingness among all groups to assume addi-tional clinical functions. ED physicians are generally receptive to this, although they disagree about some of these tasks. At a time of increasing ED patient loads and sharply rising costs, maximum utili-zation of all personnel is essential.[3]

A VIEW OF STAFFING PATTERNS USING REGRESSION ANALYSIS

We attempted to examine ED nonphysician staffing patterns using linear regression analysis. This is not an attempt to develop the ideal staffing for an emergency department but to show that Connecticut hospitals vary substantially in their ED staffing policies.[4]

The ratio of scheduled man-hours per patient visit was calculated by using patient visits for fiscal year 1970 (10/1/69–9/30/70) and staffing patterns that existed in November 1971. Each of the hospi-tal's visits and man-hours was plotted on graphs, and a "best-fit" line was developed through linear-regression techniques (see Figs. 8–1 through 8–6). Contrasting the slope of the line developed for sched-uled RN hours (Fig. 8–1, $.1807x$) with that for scheduled non-RN hours (Fig. 8–2, $.1169x$), the reliance on RN staffing is highlighted. RN hours are added at a greater rate than non-RN hours as patient visits increase, most likely because the RNs have a greater involve-ment in direct patient-care activities. Figure 8–3 shows the progres-sion of total scheduled man-hours as well as the RN and non-RN hour regression lines.

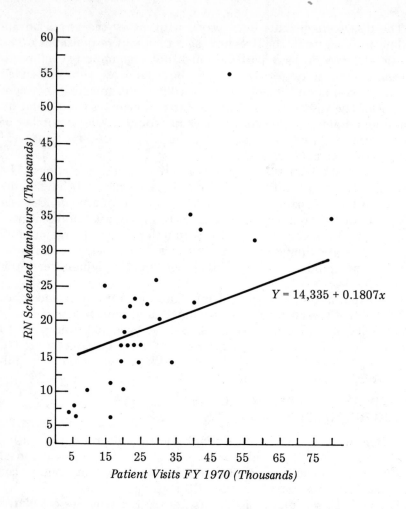

Figure 8-1. Best-fit Line for Scheduled Registered Nurse Man-Hours (reported Nov. 1971) and Number of Patient Visits, FY 1970; Connecticut Emergency Departments.

The distinct lines for RNs, non-RNs, and the progression of the two (Fig. 8–3) were subjected to cluster analysis to determine possible trends within hospitals grouped by patient visits. By grouping hospitals in categories of 0–10,000 visits, 10,000–30,000 visits, and over 30,000 visits, regression lines were developed for the staffing in each group (Figs. 8-4, 8-5, 8-6).

Through this analysis, we have substantiated that there is a wide degree of variation in staffing patterns and that the RN seems to be relied upon more heavily for patient care than other nonphysician personnel. There is a significant variation in the mix of man-hours per patient visit among hospitals experiencing a similar volume of work. The cost implications of the variations in staffing become obvious if one applies the median hourly wage for full-time RNs ($4.50) and that for full-time A/Os ($2.76) to the scheduled man-hours. In two hospitals in the over 30,000 visit category, the total scheduled

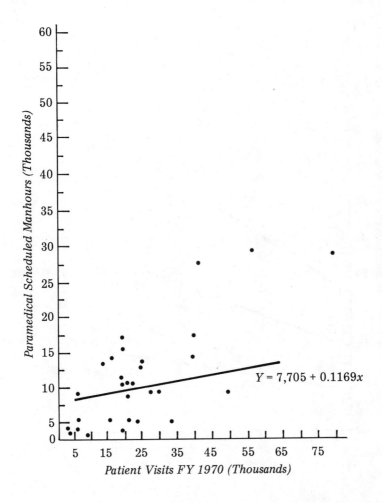

Figure 8-2. Best-fit Line for Scheduled Paramedical Man-Hours (reported Nov. 1971) and Number of Patient Visits, FY 1970; Connecticut Emergency Departments.

man-hours were less than 500 hours apart, but the salary expense differed by $35,000, primarily because of the mix of RNs and non-RN personnel. Furthermore, the hospital with lower salary expenses saw 62 percent more patients. Other factors such as diagnostic case mix are beyond the scope of this study and would have to be examined to determine which hospital was correct in its staffing policy. The

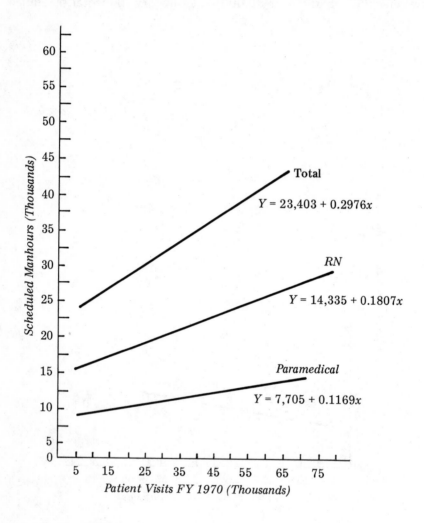

Figure 8-3. Best-fit Lines for Scheduled Man-Hours (reported Nov. 1971) and Number of Patient Visits, VY 1970; Connecticut Emergency Departments.

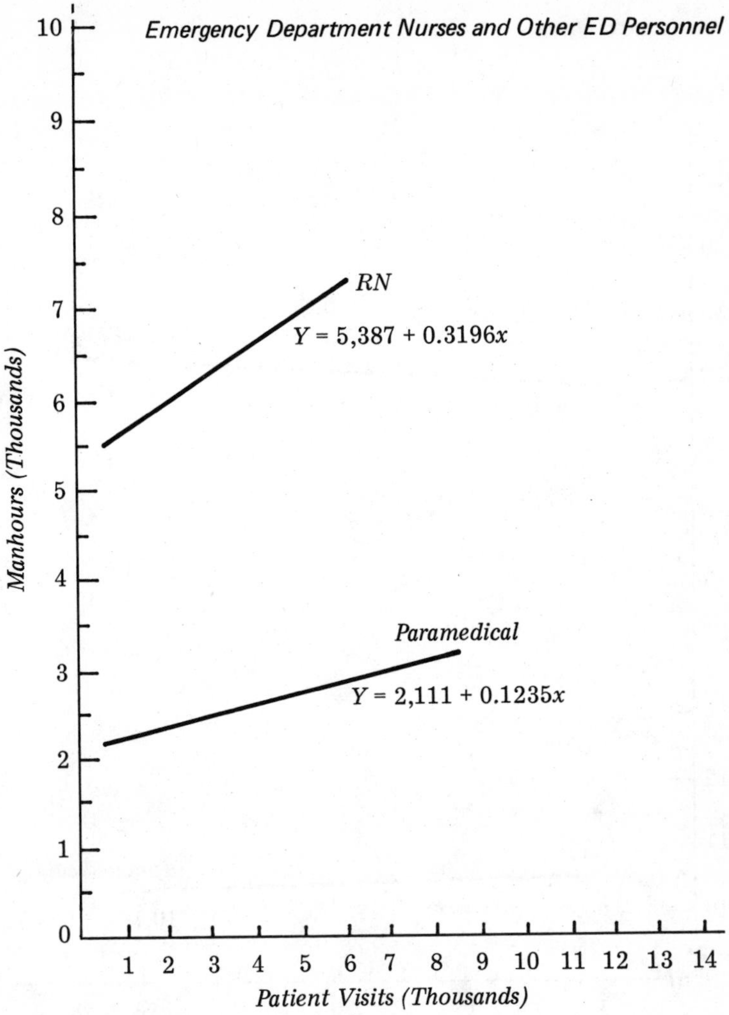

*Eight Hospitals

Figure 8-4. Linear Regression for Man-Hours and Visits, 0–10,000 Patient Visit Class Hospital Emergency Departments.*

dollar savings which might result from an analysis of proper staffing by professional category deserve careful study.

SUMMARY OF FINDINGS

The emergency department nurses and other EMS personnel studied in this chapter are predominantly young, white, and female in the

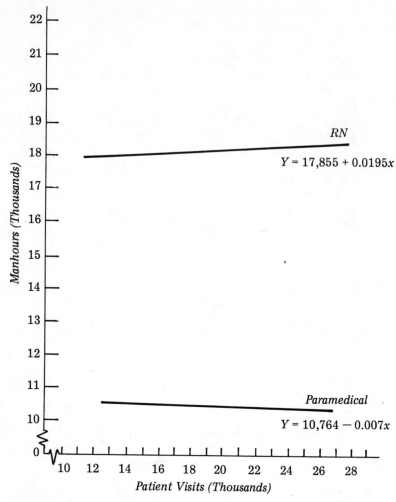

*Eighteen Hospitals

Figure 8-5. Linear Regression for Man-Hours and Visits 10,000–30,000 Patient Visit Class Hospital Emergency Departments.*

licensed professions (RNs and LPNs), and predominantly male in the others (A/Os and "other"). Nearly all ED personnel studied prefer to work in the emergency department rather than other areas of the hospital.

None of the ED personnel groups has had substantial training in emergency medical care. All personnel groups seemed to respond to the excitement and challenge associated with ED work and were enthusiastic about assuming additional tasks and enlarging their job role. ED physicians are generally receptive to this, although they disagree about some of these tasks.

Staffing patterns throughout the state varied significantly among and within classes of hospitals grouped by number of patient visits. Linear regression showed that staffing man-hours statewide varied directly with increases in patient visits. RNs are added to the staffing mix at a faster rate than other personnel as patient visits increase in the 0–30,000 visit group of hospitals.

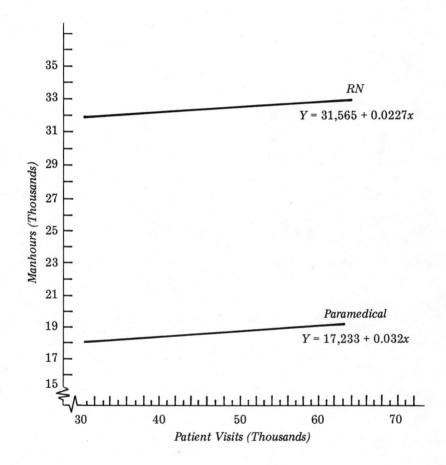

*7 Hospitals

Figure 8-6. Linear Regression for Man-Hours and Visits, Over 30,000 Patient Visit Class Hospital Emergency Departments.*

✳ *Part IV*

Improving the System

Chapter 9

Legal and Regulatory Issues

INTRODUCTION AND OBJECTIVES

The regulation of emergency medical services in Connecticut, like their organization and delivery, was fragmented, inadequate, and in some cases nonexistent at the time of the statewide study. The State Health Department had some standard-setting authority over hospital emergency departments, but most of the emergency ambulance services were completely unregulated. Although state standards for such vocations as barbers and hairdressers were clear, rigorous, and strictly enforced, there were no standards for most ambulance services relating to training, vehicles, equipment, or availability.

In addition, myths abounded about the legal ramifications of delivering emergency care. An example was the impression that physicians or others were likely to be successfully sued for malpractice if they provided care at the emergency scene or that ambulance attendants were subject to legal risk for "practicing medicine" without a license if they performed anything beyond the most basic first-aid procedures.

We explored these issues through a detailed review of legislation, regulations, and judicial decisions of other states, and through discussions with legal experts. This chapter contains our observations based on this review but is not intended to be a comprehensive analysis of every area where the law relates to emergency care. Instead we focused on those areas directly relevant to developing a coordinated system of emergency care in Connecticut. These areas include ambulance services, persons delivering emergency care, and hospital emergency departments.[1]

AMBULANCE SERVICES

Ambulance services in Connecticut were virtually unregulated until 1967, when a law was passed creating a nine-member Connecticut State Ambulance Commission. Legislation enacted in 1969 reduced the membership to five, and 1971 legislation reduced it to four. Under the 1971 law, commercial ambulance services were regulated by the commission, which had jurisdiction over licensing and operation of commercial ambulance services, certification of ambulance technicians and drivers, and the establishment of standards for ambulance equipment. Legally, an ambulance service was defined as "an organization, the purpose of which is transporting patients in ambulances for hire." Thus, the commission's authority did not apply to volunteer, municipal, or hospital-based services, which remained completely unregulated.

Commission members were appointed by the governor and represented the Commissioner of Health, the Commissioner of Motor Vehicles, the State Police Commissioner, and the commercial ambulance services. The Health Department had authority to inspect ambulance equipment, records, and credentials, but rarely did so because of the lack of funds or personnel. The commission had authority to license commercial ambulance technicians, drivers, and instructors, but this had not been done.[a]

The commission also had authority to revoke or suspend a license, and the law required that all vehicles be equipped with a "two-way radio communications system."[b] The law further required that trip logs be kept of each ambulance run, but no required (or even suggested) forms had been developed, and this requirement was never enforced. This helped to explain our difficulty in obtaining even the most basic ambulance data.

Interestingly, the state's Public Utilities Commission (PUC) had jurisdiction over setting rates for commercial ambulance services. Although the law required the PUC to "exercise its powers . . . with

---

[a]In May, 1973, as a result of stimulus from the Connecticut Advisory Committee on EMS, the commission issued regulations stating that as of January 1, 1974, all such drivers or attendants would have to be graduates of the eighty-one-hour EMT course (see Chapter 11).

[b]This in part explains the high percentage of vehicles with two-way radios discussed in Chapter 4, although, as that analysis shows, most radio communications capability was limited to the ambulance driver and his dispatcher.

respect to such matters only after consultation with the Ambulance Commission," the commission provided little guidance for the PUC in establishing fair and equitable rates, and, as Chapter 5 shows, there were no reliable data on the actual costs of providing ambulance services. Thus rates were set on an individual service basis, and there was considerable disparity between rates authorized in different parts of the state. Rarely was there an opportunity for consumers (or anyone but the applicant service) to present even the crudest information regarding the quality or accessibility of service.

Any person or town had legal authority to make a written complaint to the commission regarding deficiencies in ambulance service, in which case the commission would hold hearings and impose sanctions (with a maximum $400 fine or thirty days imprisonment for each offense). The commission held regular meetings and attempted to carry out the law. But because of the incomplete scope of the statute (which applied only to commercial services) and the lack of budget and staff, its impact was limited. Criticism of ambulance services was commonplace, competition for patients existed in certain areas, and allegations of fraud were made in several instances.

PERSONS DELIVERING EMERGENCY CARE

Laws concerning individuals delivering emergency medical care are of two types—criminal and civil. Criminal laws relate to the issue of licensure and the authority to practice; civil laws to malpractice and liability for negligent acts.

Licensure and the Authority to Practice

According to Chapter 370 of the Connecticut Medical Practice Act, "No person shall, for compensation, gain or reward . . . diagnose, treat, operate or prescribe for any injury, deformity, ailment or disease . . . of another person, nor practice surgery until he has obtained a certificate of registration. . . ."[2] Historically, this definition of the practice of medicine in Connecticut has been applied only to the licensed physician. This might give rise to the concern that an emergency medical technician or other individual rendering emergency care could be held responsible for violating the Act by "practicing medicine" without a license. However, the Act makes an exception for such cases by stipulating that its prohibitions do not apply to "any person who furnishes medical or surgical assistance in cases of sudden emergency."

The question of licensing the emergency medical technician (EMT) comes at a time when licensure of all health professions is under heavy attack. Enacted in the nineteenth century to protect the public from quacks and incompetent practitioners, licensure laws are now viewed as unnecessary barriers to educational advancement, effective delegation of tasks, and innovation in manpower utilization. Furthermore, they have failed to solve the problems of the incompetent and unethical practitioner.[3] These conclusions, which appeared in position statements on licensure prepared in 1970 by the AMA and the AHA, are consistent with the views of most scholars in the field.[4] A Department of Health, Education and Welfare report to Congress on licensure and related health-personnel credentialing issued in June 1971 reached the same conclusion and joined with the previous statements in urging a moratorium on licensure of additional health occupations.[5]

In lieu of licensure, the Advisory Committee on EMS favored the development of a certification examination of competency that could eventually be linked to the national registry for EMTs. Once the test is developed and validated, one might be able to be certified as an EMT by passing the test without having to take the eighty-one-hour course if previous work experience can be shown.

When training progresses to the EMT-II or paramedic level, additional questions arise, in part because there is no uniformity of program length, type or content at the advanced level. Many EMT-II responsibilities (e.g., starting an IV or giving drugs) contain considerable risks if performed improperly and should only be done under the supervision of a physician. The physician need not be physically present to provide such supervision if two-way voice communications capability exists, and standing orders or protocols can be used. To permit this type of functioning by remote supervision, the Connecticut Medical Practice Act was amended in 1972 to permit "services rendered by a physician's trained assistant, a registered nurse or licensed practical nurse if such services are rendered under the supervision, control and responsibility of the licensed physician."[6] This flexible provision allows for experimentation and the evolution of new types of health professionals such as physician assistants and advanced EMTs, while still protecting the public through the requirement of physician supervision and responsibility.

Liability

Generally, an individual is held legally responsible for the delivery of health care on the basis of his experience and training. However, considerable controversy has arisen over the question of liability when an individual (whether he is a physician or not) renders care at the scene of an accident. Because of the increasing number of malpractice verdicts and the size of the monetary awards, it is understandable that many health professionals are concerned that stopping to help in such a case might lead to a malpractice suit. But this is not a well-founded fear because the law permits a flexible standard of care according to the circumstances. Consequently, a physician is not held to the same standard of care in a roadside emergency as in a hospital operating room or his own office. An AMA study undertaken in 1965 indicated that only eight physicians had ever been sued for malpractice in good Samaritan situations, and all these suits were settled in favor of the physician.[7] Since that time, we are aware of no successful lawsuit concerning the rendering of care in good Samaritan settings.

In spite of these facts, most states have enacted good Samaritan statutes to provide immunity from liability for emergency medical assistance or first aid. In 1969, the following provision was enacted in Connecticut under Section 52-557(b):

No ... licensed ... physician, no person licensed as a registered nurse or licensed practical nurse ... who, voluntarily and gratuitously and other than in the ordinary course of his employment or practice, renders emergency medical or professional assistance to a person in need thereof, and no paid or volunteer fireman or policeman, and no ambulance personnel, which firemen, policemen, or ambulance personnel has completed a course in first aid offered by the American Red Cross, the American Heart Association, the State Department of Health or any other municipal health department, as certified by the agency offering such course, who renders emergency first aid to a person in need thereof, shall be liable to such person assisted for civil damages for any personal injuries which result from acts or omissions by such person in rendering the emergency care or first aid, which may constitute ordinary negligence. This immunity does not apply to acts or omissions constituting gross, willful or wanton negligence.

Therefore, none of these individuals (including EMTs who are graduates of a course sponsored by the state Health Department) can be held liable for ordinary negligence; their acts or omissions must be found by a court to constitute "gross, willful or wanton negligence." We are not aware of any lawsuits in Connecticut that have been brought against individuals for rendering emergency medical assistance.

In short, legal liability does not appear to be a real problem for adequately trained individuals rendering EMS. Good training and preparation are the best defenses against a lawsuit. As the result of the "good Samaritan" law, the legal standard in Connecticut is liberal, since even ordinary negligence produces no liability. Fear of malpractice should not, therefore, be a deterrent to rendering emergency medical care in the state.

REGULATION OF HOSPITAL EMERGENCY DEPARTMENTS

Section 19 of the Connecticut Public Health Code contains provisions concerning the regulation of Connecticut hospitals by the state Health Department. Section 19-13-D3(j) required all hospitals to prepare for emergencies as follows.

> Provision shall be made to maintain essential services during disaster and similar emergency situations. Each general hospital shall be organized in such a way as to provide adequate care for persons with acute emergencies at all hours.

However, subsection (j) was amended in 1971 to provide:

> In a city or town with two or more hospitals, the operation by one such hospital, under a mutual agreement, acceptable to the Connecticut state department of health, of an emergency room twenty-four hours a day shall be considered satisfactory compliance with this section; in other hospitals arrangements shall be made to operate an emergency room twenty-four hours a day with a physician to be available within twenty minutes of the call to the physician.

This amendment recognizes that hospitals could participate in a categorization plan such as that discussed in Chapters 6, 10, and 11 and adequately serve the public.

SUMMARY OF FINDINGS

There is no legal structure that gives any agency comprehensive authority or responsibility for planning, developing, evaluating, and regulating emergency medical services in the state. Commercial ambulance services are subject to some minimum state standards but they are rarely enforced, and municipal and volunteer services are completely unregulated.

The Connecticut Medical Practice Act provides flexible authorization for various health personnel to perform certain procedures while acting under physician supervision, control, and responsibility, and the state's good Samaritan legislation provides considerable protection from liability in emergency settings. The state Health Department has authority to set standards for hospital emergency departments and hospitals are able to participate in a categorization plan through mutual agreements under the law.

※ *Chapter 10*

Selected Findings, Recommendations, and Statement of Priorities

This chapter begins with a summary of the major study findings presented in Chapters 3 through 9 based on data collected in 1971. The recommendations we made in 1972 for improving EMS in Connecticut follow. The chapter concludes with a statement of priorities, assignment of responsibility, and a schedule for implementation.

SELECTED STUDY FINDINGS

Emergency Ambulance Services

Connecticut's ambulance vehicles make, on the average, only one trip per day.

On an average, there is one ambulance call per 11,000 people per day.

Forty-two percent of the ambulance services made between 50 and 250 trips during 1970—significantly less than one per day.

The 141 Connecticut ambulance services surveyed provide emergency coverage to a total area two times the size (in square miles) of the state.

Based on U.S. Department of Transportation (DOT) criteria, there are no significant differences between commercial, volunteer, and municipal services in Connecticut.

Overall compliance with DOT standards by Connecticut emergency ambulance services is clearly below par. For instance, only 22 percent of all services require an Advanced Red Cross certificate before they will hire a driver-attendant.

Performance is also poor in terms of emergency vehicles and equipment. Only three purveyors carry the six "essential" rescue items recommended by the American College of Surgeons on all emergency vehicles, and none of the services carries both the essential first aid supplies and medical equipment *and* the rescue equipment items.

Nearly half of the ambulance purveyors could not provide an accurate account of the total number of runs made per year, or information regarding the type of calls.

Of those services keeping records, approximately one-third of all calls were for routine transportation rather than emergency purposes.

Fifty ambulance services have no listing in any telephone book.

Twelve ambulance services dispatch a vehicle manned by only one driver/attendant.

The clear need for improvement is highlighted by the fact that not one ambulance service meets all the criteria approved by the National Highway Traffic Safety Administration of the U.S. Department of Transportation.

Emergency Medical Communications

In most communities, there is no well-publicized number to call to request emergency medical assistance.

In several communities, a citizen cannot obtain an ambulance unless the request has first been "verified" by a policeman who is dispatched to the scene. In several other communities, a fire rescue vehicle is dispatched to render first aid and then determine if an ambulance is needed to transport the patient. In both cases, valuable life-saving time may be lost.

Although the Presidential Commission on Civil Disorders recommended in 1968 the establishment of 911 as a single emergency telephone number and the American Telephone and Telegraph Company announced its availability in that year, only fourteen such 911 systems have been established in Connecticut serving only 14 percent of the population.

Fifty percent of the police and fire agencies that are called for emergency medical assistance relay the call to another agency.

Although 55 percent of Connecticut towns reported central dispatching of two or more emergency services (police/fire/ambulance/rescue), 87 percent of these were in single town (rather than regional) areas. In approximately 90 percent of the cases, the fire department performed this central dispatching function.

Although 73 percent of the hospitals have two-way radio equipment and all but three ambulance companies have two-way radio equipment linking their dispatcher and vehicles, only 5 percent of the ambulance vehicles can communicate *directly* by radio with hospital emergency departments.

Costs of Ambulance Services

The average cost per run for ambulance service is: commercial, $33.45; volunteer, $21.73; and municipal, $46.72. (The municipal figure is higher largely as a result of higher salary costs which include fringe benefits. The volunteer figure is lower largely because of donated time.)

The estimated cost *per person per year for ambulance service* is $1.66 in the service area studied. This compares favorably with annual costs for police and fire protection, which in one town, were $25 and $19 per person, respectively.

Over 20 percent of ambulance calls that are billed are not paid. Of these, more than half result from service provided to nonresidents of the service area.

Approximately one-fifth of all ambulance purveyors received monetary subsidies in 1970 and one-third received monetary-equivalent subsidies in free goods and services during that year.

Hospital Emergency Departments

The utilization of Connecticut hospital emergency departments increased in patient visits by 262 percent from 1960 to 1974.

Compared to information reported from most other states, Connecticut hospital emergency departments measure up rather well. They also measure up rather well when compared to other elements of EMS in Connecticut.

All thirty-five emergency departments provide some form of medical coverage twenty-four hours a day and the majority have physician specialists on call around the clock.

Most EDs maintain the recommended resuscitation equipment and "emergency trays" necessary for lifesaving therapy. However, some share equipment (defibrillators, electrocardiographs, and cardioscopes) with other hospital departments.

While all EDs are guided by written policies and procedures, deficiencies were noted regarding the policies required by the Joint Commission on Accreditation of Hospitals.

All thirty-five hospitals reported having a general intensive care unit and three-fourths have an additional coronary care unit functioning twenty-four hours a day.

Substantial emergency department construction and overhaul is in progress, indicating a responsiveness of the hospitals to meet increased utilization.

Only 48 percent of Connecticut emergency departments provide for the separation of the critically ill from nonurgent patients.

Some hospitals have emergency patients brought to their emergency departments by commercial purveyors on a rotating basis without regard to the proximity and availability of the ambulance.

Most ambulances transport the patient to the nearest hospital rather than to the facility best equipped to treat the patient.

Emergency Department Physicians

One of the most striking features of ED physician manpower is its organizational diversity. Ten different staffing patterns exist, and not one is common to a majority of the hospitals.

Nearly two-thirds of the hospitals utilize salaried ED-based physicians in covering their emergency departments, a threefold increase during the past five years.

The majority of full-time ED physicians are from ages forty-one to fifty-five, thus indicating that they did not "retire" to emergency medical work.

Most full-time ED physicians move into this work from private practice in midcareer and from the immediate vicinity of the hospital. Their principal reason for making the change is predictability of working hours. Part-time ED physicians cite income advantages as their principal attraction.

Nearly all full-time ED physicians expect to remain in ED work.

Nearly 45 percent of the full-time emergency department physicians indicated they had not participated in a postgraduate course in emergency medical care.

Nine out of ten physicians expressed an interest in attending a postgraduate program in emergency care, yet less than a quarter of the institutions offered any continuing-education programs for physicians.

Training in cardiopulmonary resuscitation and in the management of pediatric emergencies were listed by physicians as topics of greatest interest.

Emergency Department Nurses and
Other ED Personnel

Nearly all ED personnel studied prefer to work in the emergency department rather than other areas of the hospital.

None of the ED personnel groups has had substantial training in emergency medical care.

Only 46 percent of the nurses working in the emergency department have received any special training in emergency care.

All personnel groups seemed to respond to the excitement and challenge associated with ED work and were enthusiastic about assuming additional tasks and enlarging their job role. ED physicians are generally receptive to this, although they disagree about some of these tasks.

Ninety-six percent of emergency department nurses indicated they would take additional training if offered at hospital expense and 48 percent indicated they would take the additional training even if offered at their own expense.

Staffing patterns varied significantly among and within classes of hospitals grouped by number of patient visits. Linear regression showed that staffing man-hours statewide varied directly with increases in patient visits.

Legal and Regulatory Issues

There is no legal structure that gives any agency comprehensive authority or responsibility for planning, developing, evaluating, and regulating emergency medical services in the state.

Commercial ambulance services are subject to some minimum state standards but they are rarely enforced, and municipal and volunteer services are completely unregulated.

The Connecticut Medical Practice Act provides flexibility for various health personnel to perform certain procedures while acting under physician supervision, control, and responsibility, and the state's good Samaritan legislation provides considerable protection from liability in emergency settings.

The state Health Department has authority to set standards for hospital emergency departments and hospitals are able to participate in a categorization plan through mutual agreements under the law.

RECOMMENDATIONS

Emergency Ambulance Services

1. As soon as feasible, all ambulance driver/attendants should be certified or licensed by the state of Connecticut. To qualify, applicants should fulfill such minimum requirements as:

a. At least eighteen years of age.
b. A driver's license issued by the Motor Vehicle Department of the state of Connecticut.
c. A good driving record—no more than three convictions for traffic violations within the past five years.
d. No serious police record, i.e., felony.
e. Ability to speak, read, and write the English language.
f. Annual medical examination by a physician licensed by the state of Connecticut.

2. Given availability of the Emergency Medical Technician I (EMT-I) course, plus adequate instructor training, no person should be employed to serve as an ambulance driver/attendant unless at the time of application for employment he has completed the recognized EMT-I course, and has a valid certificate attesting to the completion of such course, or has demonstrated equivalent capability by passing a test developed for this purpose. This requirement should be mandated by law by January 1, 1975.

3. The statewide program of EMT-I training courses should continue under the sponsorship of the state Health Department and the proposed Council on Emergency Medical Services in each of the ten health service regions.

4. The state Health Department and the proposed Council on Emergency Medical Services should institute an on-going evaluation program of EMT-I graduates.

5. Comprehensive in-service training programs should be offered regularly by each ambulance organization.

6. Each vehicle utilized as an emergency ambulance should be licensed by the state of Connecticut for that purpose and fulfill such minimum requirements as:

a. Age—preferably less than five years old. Older vehicles that are otherwise adequate could be approved.
b. Design—must comply with the current DOT National Highway Traffic Safety Act Ambulance Design Criteria.

c. First Aid Supplies and Medical Equipment—must comply with the items currently recommended by the American College of Surgeons, Committee on Trauma.
d. Rescue Equipment—must comply with the items currently recommended by the American College of Surgeons, Committee on Trauma.
e. Communications—must have a two-way radio. As soon as feasible, all vehicles should have radios that can communicate with hospital emergency departments as well as ambulance dispatchers.

7. The state Health Department should regularly inspect all emergency vehicles to assure adequate health, safety, and sanitation.

8. All vehicles and driver/attendants should be covered by adequate liability insurance.

9. Purveyors should inspect their vehicles for malfunction regularly and should inspect first aid supplies and medical equipment after each run.

10. Each ambulance service should be required to keep minimum information on each ambulance run, to include such items as:

a. Patient name
b. Patient address
c. Time of receipt of emergency call
d. Time of pick-up
e. Time of discharge at the hospital
f. Hospital to which the patient is transported
g. Time of departure of the ambulance from the hospital
h. Patient's medical complaint
i. Treatment rendered by the ambulance crew
j. Type of run.

11. Each ambulance service should be required to maintain adequate records on operating costs, personnel (training, turnover rate, etc.), and vehicle equipment maintenance.

12. Management information reports should be prepared on a regular basis by each ambulance purveyor and forwarded to the state Health Department for periodic audit.

Emergency Medical Communications
1. The number 911 should be implemented as a single emergency number throughout Connecticut. Where this cannot be achieved, a

seven-digit emergency medical telephone number should be established for each community.

2. Each telephone book should contain a number for emergency medical assistance, displayed prominently with the police and fire department numbers. Telephone numbers listed as emergency medical numbers should be answered only by: (a) a person who actually dispatches emergency medical assistance; or (b) a screening operator who transfers the call directly to a dispatcher of emergency medical assistance.

3. Hospitals should have installed in their emergency departments a separate telephone with an unlisted number. It should be made known to all pertinent emergency and disaster services in the service area of the hospital.

4. Advanced clinical consultation between emergency medical service vehicles and hospital emergency departments should be established on frequencies used only for emergency medical communications.

5. The dispatch and response of ambulance services should be organized on a regional basis to improve citizen access to emergency care and to optimize effective utilization of ambulance services.

Costs of Emergency Ambulance Services

1. Communities should take responsibility for providing quality ambulance service for all their citizens without regard to their ability to pay. The cost of comprehensive ambulance services will be very low when compared with police and fire services.

2. The precedent of monetary subsidization of commercial purveyors by local governments is well established in Connecticut and should be expanded. At a minimum, commercial ambulance purveyors should be reimbursed for costs associated with dry runs and uncollectable accounts.

3. Before a cost reimbursement program can be developed, ambulance purveyors must significantly improve their record-keeping of financial operations and patterns of service. Allowable items of operational expenses must be identified and accounted for by all purveyors.

4. There is evidence to indicate that current reimbursement for emergency ambulance service under Medicare and Medicaid is unduly time consuming, inefficient, and inadequate. The issue of adequate Medicare and Medicaid reimbursement for ambulance services should be investigated in depth.

5. Because our study revealed wide variations in hospital emergency department costs that bore no relationship to the size of the

emergency department, staffing patterns, the number of beds per hospital, or the number of visits per hospital emergency department, Connecticut hospitals should redesign their accounting procedures so that the true cost of ED services can be obtained.

Hospital Emergency Departments

1. In those emergency departments where new construction or overhaul is being planned, there should be provisions for designated observation beds. The need for observation beds should be examined by all hospitals not contemplating overhaul.

2. Hospitals not having directional signs and a clearly marked entrance should correct this deficiency immediately. To produce uniformity throughout the state, signs suggested by the Department of Transportation should be utilized by all hospitals.

3. In those hospitals where space will allow, treatment areas should be arranged so that critically ill patients can be treated in designated areas away from other patients.

4. All hospitals should maintain resuscitative equipment in the emergency department twenty-four hours a day. This equipment should not be allowed outside of this area and should include: defibrillator, electrocardiograph, cardioscope, tracheal intubation equipment, central venous pressure sets, oxygen, suction apparatus, thoracotomy set, and poison tray.

5. All hospitals should require that the physician on duty be present in the emergency department twenty-four hours a day. Only if a specially trained physician's associate or nurse practitioner is on duty should a physician be "on call" somewhere else in the hospital.

6. All emergency department manuals should be updated and reviewed for completeness. Manuals should contain at least those policies required by the Joint Commission on Accreditation of Hospitals, and enforcement of these policies should be rigorous.

7. All hospitals should institute a record system which allows emergency department records to be incorporated into the hospital chart and provides for immediate access to the emergency department of past patient records.

8. Periodic review and audit of emergency department records should be made by the hospital medical staff in order to upgrade and maintain quality of care there.

9. Disaster planning policies should be reviewed and updated. Trial runs should be held at least semiannually as recommended by the Joint Commission.

10. The Connecticut Hospital Association, the Connecticut Hospital Planning Commission, the Connecticut State Medical Society, and

the American College of Surgeons, Committee on Trauma, using the information contained in this report, should undertake the categorization of hospital emergency facilities. In developing a categorization plan, cognizance should be taken of physician and nonphysician staffing patterns (including specialty backup), equipment, emergency department facilities, and hospital support facilities such as the capability for neurosurgical intervention, cardiac surgery, and coronary care units.

Emergency Department Physicians

1. In addition to specialists "on-call," hospitals should designate physicians to serve as backup to insure adequate staffing in the event of a sudden influx of emergency patients.

2. All hospitals should determine the peak utilization periods in their emergency departments and arrange staffing levels to accommodate the increased patient load.

3. Those hospitals that have a very low physician man-hour per visit ratio should review the adequacy of their staffing levels with respect to their utilization.

4. The coverage of the emergency department by interns (if maintained) should only be performed if physical supervision of patient care can be provided with members of the senior house staff or attending staff. Coverage by junior residents (if maintained) should be performed under the active supervision of the senior house staff or attending staff physicians.

5. Not all physicians (due to the nature of their specialty) are fully competent in every aspect of emergency medical treatment. Thus, policy guidelines for consultations and referrals should be made explicit to insure appropriate patient care.

6. Each hospital should have a medical director of the emergency department whose responsibilities are consistent with the guidelines of the American College of Surgeons, Committee on Trauma. This physician should act as the chairman of the emergency department committee which should serve in an advisory capacity.

7. Each hospital should have an emergency department committee consisting of members of the medical, nursing, and administrative staffs. The committee should address such issues as:

a. Determining the operational policies of the emergency department

b. Developing methods for improving the delivery of emergency care

c. Coordinating staff educational programs in the medical management of emergency patients

d. Reviewing a sample of emergency medical records as an adjunct to the hospital's utilization review, medical audit, or patient care studies committees.

8. All hospitals should support continuing education programs for all patient care personnel working in the emergency department. Although the exact nature of the programs should be determined by the emergency department committees, strong emphasis should be placed on cardiac resuscitation and major trauma management.

Emergency Department Nurses and Other ED Personnel

1. The job role of the registered nurse should be expanded to allow more opportunity to assess the patient's requirements (triage) and to take preliminary measures designed to aid the flow of work, i.e., order X-rays, do bloodwork, and assign patient priorities.

2. The role for an emergency department nurse at the nurse practitioner level should be defined. The tasks assigned to this nurse can be substantial, e.g., suturing, debridement, independent decisions regarding defibrillation, giving some medications. The relationship of this expanded nursing role to the newly developed physician's associate should be explored.

3. The physician's associate as trained at the Yale University School of Medicine, for example, can assume a range of tasks and decision-making previously allowed only the physician. These new professionals will work legally under the supervision and control of licensed physicians and should do much to expand and improve the care of patients. Their function in Connecticut emergency departments should be encouraged.

4. All emergency department personnel should receive on-going in-service training in emergency care.

Legal and Regulatory Issues

1. Recognizing that there are no state standards for ambulance services unless they are "rendered for hire," and recognizing that the current ambulance commission is understaffed and underfunded, and recognizing the need for improved coordination and organization of complex emergency medical services, there should be created the Connecticut Council on Emergency Medical Services. The council should have the authority to set overall policy and priorities relating to all aspects of emergency medical services in Connecticut. As part

of this authority, the council should develop standards and adopt regulations to carry out the policies they develop. The council should provide local and regional groups with information and advice on improving emergency medical services in their regions. The council should advise the governor through the Department of Health, the Department of Transportation, and other appropriate agencies and should make recommendations concerning the expenditure and use of all federal and state funds relating to emergency medical services. The council should have the authority to hear appeals from decisions reached by the Office of Emergency Medical Services (see recommendation 2 below). The council should develop appropriate guidelines for the establishment and coordination of regional emergency medical services councils (see recommendation 3 below).

The council should contain representatives from all appropriate groups involved in emergency medical care including physicians, hospitals, ambulance purveyors, nurses, police, fire, Red Cross, civil defense, medical schools, health planning agencies, and the public. Appointments to the council should be made by the governor for a three-year term from panels submitted to the governor by each of the groups involved.

2. An office of Emergency Medical Services should be created in the Connecticut State Health Department. The new office would operate under a full-time director of Emergency Medical Services appointed by the commissioner of health in consultation with the Council on Emergency Medical Services. The office of Emergency Medical Services would have continuing responsibility for carrying out such functions as assigned to it by the Connecticut Council on Emergency Medical Services. It is assumed such functions would include licensing and certifying ambulance personnel, enforcing standards of ambulance equipment and vehicle design, inspecting ambulances, handling consumer complaints, investigating accidents involving ambulances, and making recommendations to the Health Department's Division of Hospitals and Medical Care concerning standards for hospital emergency departments.

3. Because quality emergency medical services can be delivered in a variety of ways, each region should have the authority to develop details of emergency medical care delivery in its region. Thus, emergency medical service regions should be created consistent with the health service regions established by the state Health Department. Each region should have an Emergency Medical Services Council composed of at least one representative from all appropriate groups involved in emergency medical care, including physicians, hospitals, ambulance purveyors, the Red Cross, civil defense, and health plan-

ning agencies. Emergency Medical Services Councils should develop detailed plans for the coordination and delivery of emergency medical care in their regions and evaluate the effectiveness of their emergency medical care. Regional councils should have authority to apply for federal or state funds to improve emergency medical services in their regions. Regional councils should have the authority to recommend the imposition of tax monies in their region for the support of improved emergency medical services.

4. Currently, several Connecticut organizations are involved with the transfer of wheelchair patients, convalescents, infirm and handicapped people, and elderly individuals to and from hospitals and medical clinics. Although these are not emergency patients, they are at some medical risk. Today, there are no standards concerning the transfer of such patients to hospitals or medical clinics. The proposed Connecticut Council on Emergency Medical Services should develop appropriate standards to cover the transfer of these patients.

5. Since there is considerable duplication of ambulance services in Connecticut, it is questionable whether additional ambulance services should be established without some review of the necessity for such services. The proposed Connecticut Council on Emergency Medical Services should explore the possible applicability of need and necessity requirements to the ambulance field.

STATEMENT OF PRIORITIES

Because all recommendations cannot be acted upon at once or with equal effectiveness, we developed a ranked order of priorities. These were discussed in detail at meetings of the Connecticut Advisory Committee on EMS in September and October 1972. Suggested amendments were incorporated and the following statement of priorities was approved by the full Advisory Committee in November 1972. As such, they constituted the Committee's (as well as the study team's) blueprint for improving emergency medical services in Connecticut. In addition to priorities, they also contained a projected time frame and an assignment of responsibility to carry out the objectives. The Committee's priorities, as written November 1972, follow:

Priority No. 1. Staffing the Connecticut
Advisory Committee on EMS
At the outset, the Committee recognizes the need for staff support to increase its own effectiveness and to adequately carry out its current job. Consequently, the Committee places initial priority on the

selection and hiring of a staff director and secretary to begin on January 1, 1973. The staff director would organize and administer the future activities of the Committee as well as those of the many subcommittees that have developed. In addition, the staff director would be responsible for developing important linkages with various components of the emergency medical services system and to inform all appropriate groups of the conclusions and recommendations of the study. He would be available to meet with regional representatives to discuss how recommendations could be implemented.

The Committee also recommends support for an administrative assistant/secretary to Mr. Marshall Frankel in the Health Department to assist in the coordination and administration of the numerous emergency medical technician courses throughout the state.

Priority No. 2. Release of EMS Study and Adoption of Recommended EMS Legislation

The second major priority is the appropriate release of the Emergency Medical Services study and implementation of suggested EMS legislation. This requires informing the governor's staff, Department of Transportation officials, and all relevant groups, and the preparation of a public announcement in February 1973. In addition, legislation must be developed to create the Connecticut Council on Emergency Medical Services, the Office of Emergency Medical Services within the Health Department, and the ten regional Emergency Medical Services planning districts. The Advisory Committee will be involved in developing suggested legislation and will discuss it with appropriate groups.

Priority No. 3. Develop EMS Record and Reporting Systems

The need to develop a comprehensive emergency medical services' record and reporting system is given next priority. Eventually, this would lead to a standard form and record system used by all ambulance drivers and attendants on every run; by all emergency department personnel on every patient that was brought in; and finally, by central dispatchers who would keep a record of every call for emergency medical assistance that they receive.

Priority No. 4. Training and Public Education

The Committee places high priority on several projects. The first involves continuing the administration of the Emergency Medical Technician course until it has been completed by all ambulance drivers and attendants in Connecticut. This course will continue to be administered by the Health Department with advice from the Committee and will be held in hospitals and community colleges throughout the state.

Second, rescue training for emergency medical technicians and police and fire personnel is clearly needed. A course for instructors and for EMS personnel will be given in 1973, and will continue thereafter. This course will be organized by the State Fire Coordinator.

Third, refresher courses for EMTs are planned to begin in 1973. These courses will be given on a regular basis to all EMTs and will be administered by the Health Department.

Fourth, the need for a "first response" course for all police and fire personnel is recognized. Because all police and fire personnel will not be able to take the full eighty-one-hour EMT course, a shorter version should be prepared so that such personnel could handle an emergency situation until an EMT arrived.

Fifth, the need for continuing and special education courses for physicians and nurses in emergency medical care is recognized. The Connecticut State Medical Society, the Connecticut Chapter of the American College of Emergency Physicians, the Connecticut Nurses' Association, and the American College of Surgeons should all be involved in such courses.

Sixth, a course for ambulance dispatchers is needed. A course has been developed by the U.S. Department of Transportation for use throughout the country. The Health Department should give such a course when regional emergency medical communications networks are developed and full-time dispatchers are utilized.

Seventh, all emergency medical technicians should be tested and certified or licensed.

Eighth, the effectiveness of training of EMTs should be evaluated to determine the effect on patient care and whether the current EMT course should be modified.

The Committee also recognizes the need for public education in emergency medical services. The Connecticut Heart Association has launched a widespread effort to give CPR courses to large numbers of Connecticut citizens. The Committee believes that the Health Department, working with the Heart Association, the Red Cross, and various civic groups, should develop and help administer such courses. The effectiveness of these courses should be evaluated.

Priority No. 5. Emergency Medical Communications

The fifth major priority determined by the Committee is the need to improve emergency medical communications. The need for an adequate telephone listing for all ambulance services should be resolved without delay. The Committee places high priority on the need to develop regional emergency medical communications systems throughout Connecticut. These would include a single access number for all members of the public to call (possibly 911) and a central medical dispatcher who would have knowledge of all ambulances in the area and emergency department patient loads. The Committee also believes that local and regional EMS councils will be instrumental in the development of such systems and the EMS task force on communications will be involved in this regard. The Committee also recognizes the importance of improved clinical communications between ambulances and hospital emergency departments and the need for repeater communication systems. Finally, the Committee is aware of the need for improved communications hardware, including radios. However, the Committee believes that funds should not be used for the purchase of communications hardware until the other communications priorities have been met. The purchase of hardware without being part of an overall system would not materially improve care.

Priority No. 6. Upgrade Medical Supplies, Equipment, and Ambulance Vehicles

The sixth priority is to upgrade emergency medical supplies, equipment, and ambulances. For such items to be supported by public funds, they should comply with minimum standards on approved lists developed by the Department of Transportation and the Joint Commission on Accreditation of Hospitals.

Priority No. 7. Develop Categorization Plan for Hospital Emergency Departments

The seventh priority is to develop a categorization system of hospital emergency services. The Committee believes that all emergency departments cannot be equipped to handle all emergencies. Thus, hospital emergency services should be categorized and made part of a series of regional EMS systems. It is hoped that the Connecticut Hospital Association, the Connecticut Hospital Planning Commission, the state Medical Society, and the American College of Surgeons, Committee on Trauma, would take the leadership in this important major effort during the next three years.

Priority No. 8. Future System Development, Research, and Funding

The eighth priority is for future system development and research in emergency medical services. Such developments, including advanced training for emergency medical technicians and improved technology (including telemetry) are seen as needed, but less urgently than the other priorities presented above.

Capital and operations costs of ambulance services will continue to be provided largely through fees charged to consumers and through private donations and subscriptions. In addition, U.S. Department of Transportation money is potentially available for subsidies to ambulance services and the local tax base could be utilized for further support. It is hoped that federal and state funds will continue and will also be available to staff regional emergency medical services councils as they are developed.

Table 10-1 displays the priorities for emergency medical services in Connecticut developed by the study team and approved by the Advisory Committee.

Table 10–1. Priorities for Improving Emergency Medical Services in Connecticut

(The following EMS system components appear in the order of priority developed by the Study team and approved by the Connecticut Advisory Committee on Emergency Medical Services on November 2, 1972.)

EMS System Goals	Time Phase	Sequence of Events	Responsible Agency
I. Increase Effectiveness of Advisory Committee on EMS			
a) Hire staff director and secretary	12/15/72	Select and hire staff director and secretary to begin work 1/1/73	EMS Committee
b) Hire administrative support to Health Department to assist in EMT courses	2/1/73	Select and hire administrative assistant and secretary to begin work 2/1/73	EMS Committee Health Department
II. Release of EMS Study and Implementation of EMS Legal Structure	1972–73		
a) Inform governor's staff, DOT, and all relevant groups (including legislature)	2/1/73	Inform governor's staff, DOT, and all relevant groups	Study Team
b) Press release and public announcement	2/28/73	Press release	Study Team and EMS Committee
c) Develop legislation providing for Council on EMS, Department of EMS within Health Department and 10 Regional EMS Councils	2/28/73	Draft legislation and public hearings	EMS Committee and Legislature
III. Develop EMS Record and Reporting System	1972–74		
a) Ambulance		Legislation	EMS Committee
b) Emergency Departments		Regulations	Health Department
c) Central Dispatch		System Development	
		Cost Accounting System	

IV. Training and Public Education
   a) Training

1. Continue EMT Course until completed by all ambulance drivers and attendants	1972–75	Administer courses	Health Department EMS Committee Hospitals Community Colleges
2. Give rescue course for EMTs, police, and fire	1973–75	Administer courses for instructors and others	Fire and Civil Defense
3. Give refresher EMT course	1973–75	Administer courses	Health Department, EMS Committee, Hospitals, and Community Colleges
4. Develop and give first response course for all police and fire personnel	1973–75	Develop and administer courses	Dunlap and Associates Health Department EMS Committee
5. Administer continuing and special education courses for physicians and nurses	1973–75	Administer courses	Conn. State Medical Society, Conn. Chapter, American College of Emergency Physicians, Conn. Nurses' Association, Conn. Hospital Association, American College of Surgeons
6. Administer dispatcher course for selected ambulance personnel	1973–75	Administer courses	Health Department EMS Committee

Table 10-1 (continued)

EMS System Goals	Time Phase	Sequence of Events	Responsible Agency
7. Test, certify, and register all EMTs	1973–75	Administer national exam	National Registry EMS Committee Health Department Conn. State Medical Society Conn. College of Surgeons
8. Evaluate effectiveness of training of EMTs	1973–75	Complete Yale-New Haven Study	EMS Committee Health Department Yale Trauma Program
b) Education 1. Basic first aid and CPR	1972–75	Administer courses	Health Department Conn. Heart Association Civic Groups
2. Evaluate	1973–75	Develop evaluation instrument	EMS Committee Health Department
V. Improve Emergency Medical Communications a) Develop telephone listing for all ambulance companies	1973 (new phone book)	Letter to telephone companies (regarding false and misleading advertising); regulatory legislation	EMS Committee Telephone Company Public Utilities Commission Health Department

b) Develop single access number and central dispatch systems	1973–75	Legislation, funding criteria, and FCC waiver	Local and Regional EMS Councils EMS Subcommittee on Communications
c) Develop clinical communications ambulance to hospital	(immediate) 1973–75	FCC waiver, legislation, and funding criteria	EMS Subcommittee on Communications Health Department Conn. Hospital Association Comprehensive Health Planning Conn. Hospital Planning Comm.
d) Communications hardware, including radios	1973–75	Public support contingent upon above priorities having been achieved	EMS Committee
VI. Upgrade Medical Supplies, Equipment, and Ambulances Vehicles a) Improve and procure medical supplies and equipment	1973–75	Minimum approved ambulance equipment list	EMS Committee Ambulance Services Health Department
b) Procure new ambulances	1974–75	DOT approved design; contingent upon meeting above priorities	EMS Committee Ambulance Services Health Department
c) Improve and procure emergency room equipment and supplies	1973–75	Approved basic list JCAH Standards	EMS Committee Health Department Conn. Hospital Association

Table 10-1 (continued)

EMS System Goals	Time Phase	Sequence of Events	Responsible Agency
VII. Develop Categorization Plan for Hospital Emergency Services	1973–75	1) review baseline information; 2) develop regional plan; 3) develop categorization criteria within regions; 4) adopt and approve	Conn. Hospital Association Conn. Hospital Planning Comm. Conn. State Medical Society Conn. Chapter, American College of Emergency Physicians Health Department American College of Surgeons
VIII. a) Future System Development, 1) EMT II 2) Advanced Technology	1974–75		EMS Committee
b) Funding Sources for EMS 1) Health Department, Office of EMS	1973–75	Enactment of legislation, Health Dept. priority	State Funds, Federal Funds, CRMP
2) EMS Programs	1971–75	Priority determinations made by EMS Committee	DOT, HSMHA, CRMP
3) Capital and Operations	1973–75	Fees; Subsidies from DOT, HSMHA, local tax, private donations, and subscriptions	
4) Staff Support—Regional EMS Councils and State EMS Committee	1973–75		CRMP, DOT and local funds

Chapter 11

Epilogue—1976

INTRODUCTION

Many health care studies suffer a fatal illness—they as-
phyxiate in the dust they collect on book shelves and have
little impact beyond the classroom. As mentioned in
Chapter 2, we believe that active involvement throughout the study
process by those responsible for implementation can help to overcome this otherwise fatal syndrome.

One way to evaluate a study's success is to review retrospectively
its impact. This chapter represents our 1976 assessment of the Connecticut EMS study in fulfilling the goals and objectives developed
in 1972 (see p. 44). Although our purpose is to be objective, we
concede that the comments which follow may reveal a level of
enthusiasm explained in part by the authors' commitment to the
study and the field.

PRIORITIES

We will focus on the ranked order of priorities submitted to and
approved by the Connecticut Advisory Committee on Emergency
Medical Services on November 2, 1972. As indicated in Chapter 10,
they constitute the Committee's (as well as the study team's) blueprint for improving Connecticut's emergency medical services.

Priority No. 1. Staffing the Connecticut
Advisory Committee on EMS

To increase the likelihood of achieving study goals, the first and immediate priority was strengthening the staff of the EMS Advisory Committee. None of the recommendations of the study would have been implemented expeditiously if the principal state body devoted to EMS was unable to dispatch its duties quickly and effectively. Accordingly, first priority was placed on selecting and hiring a full-time staff director and secretary. The staff director was charged with organizing and administering future committee activities and all sub-committee functions. The staff director was made responsible for developing the necessary linkages with the components of the EMS system and to inform all appropriate groups of the conclusions and recommendations of the study. Funds to accomplish this were obtained from the Connecticut Regional Medical Program. A staff director and secretary were hired and began work in December 1972 (the target date was January 1, 1973).

The EMS Advisory Committee needed staff support to assist in the coordination and administration of the numerous Emergency Medical Technician courses throughout the state. Funds were secured from the State Department of Transportation and an administrative assistant/secretary was hired and began work January 1, 1973 (the target date was February 1, 1973).

Priority No. 2. Release of EMS Study
and Adoption of Recommended
EMS Legislation

The next major activity was the release and proper distribution of the statewide EMS study. The two volume, 700-page study, having been fully endorsed by the EMS Advisory Committee, was submitted to the governor and State Department of Transportation in December 1972.[2] A fifty-two-page summary was prepared to inform Connecticut citizens of the goals and priorities developed by the study team and the Advisory Committee. More than 5,000 copies of the summary document, "Emergency Medical Services in Connecticut—A Blueprint for Change," were distributed throughout the state at the time the governor released the study in February 1973.[3]

The Committee also recognized that legislative consideration of the study's recommenations needed active encouragement. In March 1973, a draft bill was submitted to the Connecticut General Assembly, Joint Committee on Public Health and Safety. The bill proposed the establishment of a Connecticut Council on Emergency Medical Services, an Office of Emergency Medical Services in the state Health Department, and a series of local/regional EMS councils.

Due to time constraints, the Public Health and Safety Committee did not report on this or any other EMS bill in 1973. The momentum for change was temporarily slowed. During the next year, a color movie was produced by the Yale Trauma Program entitled *EMS in Connecticut.* This was shown throughout the state to civic organizations, municipal governments, professional societies, and on public television. At the same time, 40,000 pamphlets emphasizing the thrust of the movie were produced by the Yale Trauma Program and distributed throughout the state. The interest among Connecticut citizens for improved EMS was heightened. After considerable debate, on May 30, 1974, Governor Thomas J. Meskill signed into law Public Act No. 74-305, "The Emergency Medical Services Act of 1974," which became effective on July 1, 1974.

The Emergency Medical Services Act of 1974. The new law dissolved the volunteer Connecticut Advisory Committee on Emergency Medical Services and replaced it with a twenty-five-member panel to function as the State Emergency Medical Services Council (CAC/EMS) (Public Act 74-305). The council served in an advisory capacity to the newly created State Commission on Hospitals and Health Care. The Commission on Hospitals and Health Care is the state agency that, under another 1973 law, became responsible for controlling hospital costs. With the advice of the twenty-five-member CAC/EMS, the commission was empowered to set policy and priorities for EMS utilizing the services of the state Department of Health and the Comprehensive Health Planning (CHP) "b" agencies.

Specifically, the EMS Act charged the commission, acting with the advice of the CAC/EMS, to develop and annually update a statewide plan to coordinate delivery of EMS. The Act required that the plan contain specific goals for EMS delivery; a time frame for achievement; cost data and alternative funding sources; and performance standards for the evaluation of its goals. The commission was to conduct an annual inventory of EMS resources in the state (facilities, equipment, and personnel) to determine the need for additional services and the effectiveness of existing ones, and to review and evaluate areawide plans as well as all grant and contract applications for federal and state monies concerning EMS for conformity to policy guidelines.

The commission was authorized to establish minimum standards and regulations concerning such EMS components as communications (equipment, radio frequencies, and operational procedures), transportation (vehicle type, design, condition and maintenance, life saving equipment, and operational procedures), training (EMTs, communications personnel, fire fighters, state and local police, and others as necessary), and EMS facilities (categorization of hospital EDs regarding treatment capabilities and ancillary services). It was empowered to coordinate the training of all personnel related to EMS, develop or have developed a data collection system to ensure uniform record-keeping to follow a patient from entry through discharge from the EMS system, develop a program for public education, and establish rates for the conveyance of patients in commercial ambulance vehicles and invalid carriers.

Charged with the responsibility of assisting the commission in fulfilling these duties, the CAC/EMS members were appointed by the governor and included at least one representative from each of the following: institutions of higher education; police and fire departments; hospitals; federal agencies involved in health care; medical, nursing, and mental health professions; ambulance purveyors (including one representative from volunteer ambulance associations); third party payors; and private nonprofit service agencies and state agencies concerned with EMS.

The Act established an office of EMS within the state Department of Health to be responsible for the licensure, certification, and approval of ambulance services, ambulance drivers, EMTs and communications personnel, hospital emergency department facilities and communications facilities, and transportation equipment, and for periodic inspections of ambulance equipment, emergency facilities, and ambulances to assure that state standards are maintained. All findings were to be reported to the Commission on Hospitals and Health Care. (The full text of the law is included in Appendix 11A.)

Despite the enactment of strong enabling legislation, the advancement of EMS policy became bogged down in the commission's parliamentary proceedings and the state Health Department was hampered in enforcement. In November 1973 a new commissioner of health, Douglas L. Lloyd, M.D., with a special interest in EMS was appointed. In February 1974 a new director of Emergency Medical Services, Martin Stillman, J.D., was appointed. Stillman was formerly legal counsel to the legislative committee which wrote the 1974 EMS Act, and thus had an unusual understanding of its implications and intent. These appointments helped to facilitate the enactment of new legislation entitled The Emergency Medical Services Act of 1975 on September 22, 1975 (Public Act 75-112).

The Emergency Medical Services Act of 1975. *Under the new law, the 1974 EMS Act was amended to consolidate responsibility* *for policy-making and administration of EMS in the State Health Department. The CAC/EMS now became advisory to the commissioner of health and to the governor. As presently operating, the CAC/EMS sets policy and the director of the Office of EMS is charged with its implementation.*

This new organization of EMS is precisely what the Connecticut EMS study recommended in 1972. The 1975 EMS Act authorized the development of rules and regulations which embodied the majority of the original study's recommendations, and centralized the policy-making, planning, coordination, and administration of EMS in the state Health Department.

An important provision of the 1974 Act which remains in force is the establishment of EMS regions with an EMS coordinator and council in each of the eleven CHP "b" agency regions to plan, coordinate, and implement the state EMS system. These councils must approve EMS plans in their region and submit them to the commission for ratification. In the first year (1975), $225,000 in state funds were appropriated for the commission and $50,000 for the Office of EMS in the state Department of Health. Under the new Act, for the second year (1976), $154,000 has been appropriated for the regional programs and $109,000 for the Office of EMS.[4]

We believe that the 1975 legislation represents the most significant result of the Connecticut EMS study. Because it was developed by individuals who were also concerned with its implementation, the chances for long-term success seem bright. As written, it encompasses every issue regarded as a priority item by the EMS Advisory Committee in 1972 (see Chapter 10). These include the development of a comprehensive standard EMS record and reporting form; manpower training; public education; improvement of EMS communications; improvement of EMS supplies, equipment, and ambulances; the development of categorization and regionalization of hospital emergency services; and the recognition of the need for future systems development in EMS. (The full text of the law is included in Appendix 11B and the regulations appear in Appendix 11C.)

Priority No. 3. Develop EMS Record and Reporting Systems

As mentioned, this priority is covered by the rules and regulations of the EMS legislation. In New Haven, a common record and reporting system for ambulances has been implemented. A similar system is scheduled for implementation throughout the state by the end of 1976.

A record and reporting system for hospital emergency departments is under development. The state Office of EMS will make the final necessary changes before planned implementation by the end of 1976.

Priority No. 4. Training and
Public Education

Since 1971, 5,897 ambulance drivers and attendants have been trained as EMTs (as of June 18, 1976). The number trained annually has increased from 464 in 1972 to 1,500 in 1975. In addition, 52 paramedics (EMT-II) were trained as of 1976, and by the end of 1976, 1,244 rescue personnel will have received training in shortened "first response" programs. As of June 18, 1976, 155 emergency medical services instructors have been trained to teach ambulance personnel.

In 1975 there were thirty-four EMT refresher courses given (all EMTs are now required to take a twenty-five-hour EMT refresher course every two years); and in 1976, forty such courses are being offered. There have been two EMS dispatcher courses given and several hospitals in the state have organized courses for EMS physicians and nurses.

EMTs are presently licensed and registered after passing a state written examination and a practical examination given at various locations. A written examination has been developed for rescue personnel and guidelines for a practical examination in this area have been developed.

An Association of EMTs was formed under the stimulus of the Yale Trauma Program in the south central region to enhance continuing education of EMTs. Similar associations have been formed in the eastern and southwestern regions of the state. The Yale Trauma Program provided funding for an initial evaluation of EMT performance. Subsequently, a federal grant was obtained to enlarge this Trauma Program study and evaluate the effect of the EMT on the delivery of emergency care. Another federal grant was obtained by the Yale-New Haven Medical Center EMT Program for continuation of the basic EMT course, institution of the refresher courses, and institution of an EMT dispatcher course.

There have been a number of privately sponsored efforts in EMS education. The Yale Trauma program co-sponsored with the Connecticut Committee on Trauma of the American College of Surgeons, the Connecticut Chapter of the American College of Emergency Physicians, and the Connecticut Advisory Committee on EMS, a one-day seminar in December 1973, entitled "The Emergency Department Care of the Injured Patient." Due to the excellent response, a second seminar was held in April 1974, at the University of Connecticut under the same sponsorship on the topic of "The Emergency Treatment of Infection." In June 1974, the Yale University School of Medicine was the site for a regional symposium on "Life-Saving Measures for the Critically Injured Patient," sponsored by the American College of Surgeons. The five-day symposium was well attended and covered all aspects of trauma management.

Further educational efforts have included a twenty-week core course in trauma developed in the Yale Medical School for medical students, nursing students, physician's associate students, and house officers. An additional course on clinical management of major trauma has been offered to a limited number of medical students. It is planned that this be expanded as of September 1976 to include all medical students prior to the awarding of the medical degree.

Recognizing the needs for educational material in the Yale-New Haven Hospital's Emergency Department, the Trauma Program supported the preparation of a training manual for medical students, interns, residents, and other health personnel. The manual entitled "Diagnosis and Early Management of Trauma Emergencies—A Guide to the Emergency Service," by Robert Touloukian, M.D., and Thomas J. Krizek, M.D., has been expanded into a textbook for emergency department personnel.[5]

Presently, there are plans to establish an Emergency Medical Service Education and Evaluation Center at the Yale University School of Medicine. The objectives of the center are to train all personnel who have contact with emergency patients—including police, ambulance attendants, hospital staff, nurses, private physicians, and medical students. Core instruction, first response, and advanced courses would be offered and will be designed for a particular personnel level. An EMS instructor corps and an information resource center would be developed. A methodology to evaluate training is envisioned.

Priority No. 5. Emergency Medical Communications

The EMS Regional Councils have designated an access number for emergency medical care for their respective regions throughout the state. This appears on the front page of all telephone books next to police and fire emergency numbers. While most are still seven digit numbers, there are now forty-five communities which have "911" access numbers in operation (as compared with fourteen in 1972).

Central dispatch networks are ready for implementation in the south central, central Naugatuck Valley, Colchester, and northwestern regions. Central dispatch networks are actually operational in multitown regions in the Tolland (twelve towns), Danielson (ten towns), Windham (fourteen towns), and Norwich (nine towns) areas. In two areas of the state, advanced clinical consultation between ambulance and hospitals is ongoing and many ambulances in the state now have the capability for two-way voice communication with hospitals on VHF frequencies.

The Yale-New Haven Hospital and the Hospital of St. Raphael in New Haven received a Robert Wood Johnson Foundation Grant for a Regional Emergency Medical Communications System. This program is based on the Foundation's concepts and the study's recommendations regarding regionalization (see Chapters 1 and 4). After extensive negotiations involving ambulance services, hospitals, and local governments, the ten town regional system became operational on November 29, 1976.

Priority No. 6. Upgrade Emergency Ambulance Vehicles, Equipment, and Medical Supplies

At present, over 99 percent of the ambulances in the state conform to the rules and regulations of the new EMS legislation which adopted professionally recommended guidelines for supplies and equipment.[6] This is a significant improvement over the situation that existed in 1971, when none of the state's 200 ambulances met these standards. About 60 percent of the state's vehicles now comply with the federal government's General Services Agency requirements.

Priority No. 7. Categorize Hospital Emergency Departments

After two years of work, a subcommittee of the Connecticut Trauma Committee, American College of Surgeons, presented detailed emergency department categorization guidelines and an initial plan for categorization to the CAC/EMS. The Connecticut Trauma Committee gave each hospital an opportunity to review the plan prior to its submission to the CAC/EMS. This plan was adopted on February 6, 1976, by the CAC/EMS. The hospitals have additional opportunities to comment on their categorization status prior to inspection by the state Office of EMS commencing in the summer of 1976. (Excerpts from the categorization guidelines appear in Appendix 11D.) A subcommittee of the CAC/EMS has been formed to identify critical care units throughout the state for burns, cardiac care, trauma, neonatal care, spinal cord injuries, and psychiatric and drug related emergencies. This committee will also develop protocols to be used as the basis for transfer agreements between the various Connecticut hospitals.

Priority No. 8. Future System Development, Research, and Funding

As mentioned earlier, fifty-two advanced EMTs have already been trained. Telemetry is now in use at four sites in the state. Prior to expansion in this area, evaluation of such technology with respect to patient outcome is planned and initial work in this area is underway at three sites. Funding sources remain the major drawback to increased system development.

Research in EMS is continuing both in the general fields of epidemiology and public health and in specific biomedical areas. Following the statewide EMS study, research at Yale is being directed at subelements of the EMS system. A major review of disaster planning at the local, state, national, and international levels has been completed.[7] A new system of evaluation of diagnostic and treatment care of the trauma victim, which can be used in developing standards of care and could be applied to the peer review process envisioned in the national legislation creating Professional Standards Review Organizations (PSROs), has been initiated.[8] Currently under investigation are such topics as the impact of increased emergency room department utilization on hospital operations[9,10] and an update of the 1972 EMS study focusing particularly on staffing and training of personnel in hospital emergency departments as well as categorization of EDs.[11] The epidemiology and costs of acute spinal cord injury are being studied intensively under a five-year grant from the National Institute of Neurological and Sensory Diseases.

In biomedical research, investigation at Yale is concentrating on the etiology of decubitus ulcers resulting from acute spinal cord injuries, the field of thermal injuries, traumatic soft tissue infections, and the effectiveness of present emergency resources to decrease contamination of open wounds. These ongoing programs of research should uncover needed innovations for the treatment of trauma patients.[12]

SOME AREAS FOR CONTINUED RESEARCH

There are several EMS areas which need more research. The question of hospital emergency department costs must be studied. Present financial analytic methods are not adequate primarily because most health care cost methodologies are based on inpatient accounting procedures which in turn are geared toward maximizing third-party reimbursement.

The evaluation of EMS outcomes is another area needing extensive research.[13] Research regarding the quality of EMS care is in short supply.[14] Measurable guidelines, standards, and acceptable limits of professional competence on a diagnostic specific basis can be developed only after careful study. Some work on this is presently underway under the auspices of the Yale Trauma Program and the Division of Reconstructive and Plastic Surgery at the Yale University School of Medicine.[15] In addition, under the auspices of a three-year grant from the National Center for Health Services Research, the Yale Trauma Program, the Yale Program in Hospital Administration, and the Yale Center for Health Services Research are investigating several methodologies to develop and assess EMS outcome measures in the emergency department.

CONCLUSION

In our preface, we began by noting that the many complexities involved in emergency medical services made significant improvements difficult to achieve and slow to implement. We cautioned against looking for quick, short-term solutions and readily conceded that there were many reasonable approaches to improved emergency care, including a variety of public education and prevention programs, as well as requiring seat belts or air bags in all automobiles.

But we also deplored the lack of adequate political and organizational structures to plan and organize the many components of EMS into a true system of care, and we stressed the need to upgrade these components to at least minimum levels while developing public interest and support for improved emergency care. Since, in these respects, EMS was in the dark ages when we began our efforts in Connecticut in 1970, it is quite natural that we placed heavy emphasis on structural change (in part through sorely needed legislation) and on upgrading of components such as trained personnel, communications capabilities and emergency department resources. The data gathered, the recommendations made, the priorities set, and the timetable established all reflect this emphasis.

Naturally, it is encouraging to report the significant change that has occurred in the past four years and to observe that most of the recommendations have been adopted. Thus, we believe this study may be useful to many involved in EMS throughout the country. But this merely marks the end of the first generation of concerns—it is the end of the beginning and hardly the final word.

With an aroused public, a better understanding of the problems, many of the needed structures now in place, and increasing commitment by all levels of government, the next generation of EMS studies will have to address different and possibly even more difficult issues. Among these will be the ways in which emergency medical systems are best implemented, financed and managed, the ways they are actually used by patients, providers and the public, and an assessment of the ultimate impact such systems actually have on saving and improving people's lives.

Appendix 11A

The Connecticut Emergency Medical Services Act of 1974

PUBLIC ACT NO. 74-305
AN ACT ADOPTING THE
EMERGENCY MEDICAL SERVICES ACT OF 1974.

Be it enacted by the Senate and House of Representatives in General Assembly convened:

Section 1. (NEW) As used in this act, (a) "emergency medical service system" means a system which provides for the arrangement of personnel, facilities, and equipment for the efficient, effective and coordinated delivery of health care services under emergency conditions; (b) "comprehensive health planning agency" means any health planning agency created pursuant to section 246(b) of title 42 of the United States Code, as amended, hereinafter referred to as the "b" agency; (c) "patient" means an injured, ill, crippled, or physically handicapped person requiring assistance and transportation; (d) "ambulance" means a motor vehicle specifically designed to carry patients; (e) "ambulance service" means an organization which transports patients; (f) "commission" means the commission on hospitals and health care created pursuant to section 3 of number 73-117 of the public acts of 1973; (g) "emergency medical technician" means an individual who has successfully completed the training requirements established by the commission and has been certified by the state department of health; (h) "ambulance driver" means a person whose primary function is driving an ambulance; (i) "emergency medical technician instructor" means a person who is certified by the state department of health to teach courses, the completion of which are required in order to become an emergency medical technician; (j) "communications facility" means any facility housing the personnel and equipment for handling the emergency communications needs of a particular geographic area; (k) "life saving equipment" means equipment used by emergency medical personnel for the stabilization and treatment of patients; (l) "emergency medical service organization" means any organization whether public, private or voluntary which offers transportation or treatment services to patients under emergency conditions; (m) "invalid coach" means a vehicle used exclusively for the transportation of non-ambulatory patients to or from either a medical facility or the patient's home in non-emergency situations or utilized in emergency situations as a back-up vehicle when insufficient emergency vehicles exist; (n) "rescue service" means any organization, whether profit or nonprofit, whose primary purpose is to search for persons who have become lost or to render emergency service to persons who are in dangerous or perilous circumstances; and (o) "provider" means any person, corporation or organization, whether profit or nonprofit, whose primary purpose is to deliver medical care or services, including such related medical care services as ambulance transportation.

Sec. 2. (NEW) The commission shall be the state agency responsible for the planning, coordination and administration of a statewide emergency medical care service system. The commission with the advice of the Connecticut advisory committee on emergency medical services, as established in section 4 of this act, shall set policy and establish statewide priorities for emergency medical services utilizing the services of the state department of health and the "b" agencies and their associated emergency medical service councils, as established by section 12 of this act.

Sec. 3. (NEW) The commission shall: (a) With the advice of the Connecticut advisory committee on emergency medical services as established in section 4 of this act, develop and annually update a statewide plan for the coordinated delivery of emergency medical services, which plan shall take into account the needs of the "b" agencies. The plan shall contain: (1) Specific goals for the delivery of such emergency medical services; (2) a time frame for achievement of such goals; (3) cost data and alternative funding sources for the development of such goals; and (4) performance standards for the evaluation of such goals;

(b) Annually inventory or cause to be inventoried emergency medical services resources within the state, including facilities, equipment, and personnel, for the purposes of determining the need for additional services and the effectiveness of existing services;

(c) Review and evaluate all areawide plans developed by the "b" agencies pursuant to section 11 of this act in order to insure conformity with standards issued by the commission;

(d) Within thirty days of their receipt, review all grant and contract applications for federal or state funds concerning emergency medical services or related activities for conformity to policy guidelines and forward such application to the appropriate agency, when required.

(e) Establish such minimum standards and adopt such regulations in accordance with the provisions of chapter 54 of the general statutes, as may be necessary to develop the following components of an emergency medical service system: (1) Communications, which shall include, but not be limited to, equipment, radio frequencies and operational procedures; (2) transportation services, which shall include, but not be limited to, vehicle type, design, condition and maintenance, life saving equipment and operational procedure; (3) training, which shall include, but not be limited to, emergency medical technicians, communications personnel, para-professionals associated with emergency medical services, firefighters and state and local police; (4) emergency medical service facilities, which shall include, but not be limited to, categorization of emergency departments as to their treatment capabilities and ancillary services;

(f) Coordinate training of all personnel related to emergency medical services;

(g) Develop or cause to be developed a data collection system which shall include a method of uniform patient record keeping which will follow a patient from initial entry into the emergency medical service system through discharge from the emergency room;

(h) Develop a program for public education and information which takes into account the needs of visitors to as well as residents of the state;

(i) Establish rates for the conveyance of patients in commercial ambulance vehicles and invalid coaches provided the present rates established by the public utilities commission for such vehicles shall remain in effect until such time as the commission establishes a new rate schedule as provided herein;

(j) No later than December 31, 1975, and annually thereafter submit a report to the governor and general assembly which shall include, but not be limited to, the following: (1) An accounting of all federal and state funds expended for emergency medical services in the state; (2) a statement and evaluation of the accomplishments of the office of the statewide deputy director of emergency medical services during the preceding year together with a description of goals for the upcoming year; and (3) recommendations for any legislation which the commission feels will facilitate a complete coordinated emergency medical services system;

(k) If no "b" agency exists within a region, develop in conjunction with the regional coordinator, as established by section 14 of this act, an emergency medical services plan for such region, such plan to conform with the requirements of section 11 of this act.

Sec. 4. (NEW) (a) There is established a Connecticut advisory committee on emergency medical services which shall advise the commission regarding comprehensive emergency medical services. Said advisory committee shall be composed of twenty-five members appointed by the governor and shall include at least one representative of each of the following: (1) Institutions of higher education; (2) police and fire officials; (3) hospital representatives; (4) federal agencies involved in health care; (5) medical, nursing and mental health officials; (6) provider representation, including one representative of volunteer ambulance associations; (7) third party payors; (8) paraprofessionals; (9) private nonprofit service agencies and (10) officials of state agencies which are concerned with the emergency medical service delivery system.

(b) All members serving on the ad hoc state advisory committee on emergency medical services on the effective date of this act shall be eligible for appointment pursuant to the provisions of this section. In making such initial appointments to said advisory committee, the governor shall give consideration to (1) a list of names submitted to him by the ad hoc advisory committee on emergency medical services and (2) the goal of maintaining a balance between rural and urban communities within the state.

Sec. 5. (NEW) The commission shall appoint a deputy director for emergency medical services, who shall be the statewide emergency medical services coordinator. Such deputy director shall be in the classified service and shall be responsible for administering the duties of the commission as provided in section 3 of this act, in conformance with the policies and standards adopted by the commission.

Sec. 6. (NEW) There shall be established within the state department of health an office of emergency medical services. The office shall be responsible for (a) the licensure or certification of the following: (1) Ambulance operations, ambulance drivers, emergency medical technicians, and communications personnel; (2) emergency room facilities and communications facilities and (3) transportation equipment, including land, sea and air vehicles used for transportation of patients to emergency facilities and (b) periodic inspections of life saving equipment, of emergency facilities and of emergency transportation vehicles to insure that state standards are maintained. The office shall report its findings to the commission.

Sec. 7. (NEW) (a) There shall be a director of the office of emergency medical services as established in section 6 of this act who shall be appointed by and responsible to the commissioner of health. The director shall carry out the duties of the office of emergency medical services as provided in section 6 of this act and shall be responsible for adopting regulations concerning the methods and conditions for licensure and certification of the operations, facilities and equipment enumerated in section 6 of this act and regulations regarding complaint procedures for the public and any emergency medical service organization. Such regulations shall be adopted in accordance with the provisions of chapter 54 of the general statutes and shall be in conformity with the policies and standards established by the commission. All regulations adopted by the ambulance commission and in force at the time of passage of this act shall remain in effect until such time as new regulations concerning the methods and conditions for licensure and certification of the operations, facilities and equipment enumerated in section 6 of this act and regulations regarding complaint procedures for the public and any emergency medical service organization are adopted by the director of the office of emergency medical services in accordance with the provisions of this section.

(b) (1) The assignment or transfer of any of the functions, powers or duties of the ambulance commission under any of the provisions of this act shall not affect any action or proceeding, civil or criminal, pending at the time of such assignment or transfer, and the office of emergency medical services shall be deemed substituted in such action by operation of this subsection without motion or order. (2) Any right of action or matter undertaken or commenced by the ambulance commission, the functions, powers or duties of which are assigned or transferred, may be conducted and completed by the office of emergency medical services in the same manner and under the same terms and conditions and with the same effect as if undertaken or commenced and conducted and completed by the ambulance commission. (3) The chairman of the ambulance commission shall deliver to the office of emergency medical services, all contracts, books, maps, plans, papers, records and property pertaining to or used in connection with the functions, powers or duties assigned or transferred, to said office.

Sec. 8. (NEW) The director of the office of emergency medical services may employ, subject to the provisions to chapter 67 of the general statutes, as amended, with the approval of the commissioner of health, such staff as is necessary to carry out the responsibilities of the office provided for in this act.

Sec. 9. (NEW) (a) No person shall operate any ambulance service or rescue service without a certificate issued by the office of emergency medical services. No person shall operate a commercial ambulance or commercial rescue service without both a certificate and a license issued by the office of emergency medical services. A certificate shall be issued to any volunteer, commercial or municipal ambulance service which shows proof satisfactory to the commission, of meeting the minimum standards of the commission in the areas of training, equipment and personnel. Applicants for a license shall use the forms prescribed by the office of emergency medical services and shall submit such application to the office of emergency medical services accompanied by an annual fee of one hundred dollars. Each applicant for licensure shall furnish proof of financial responsibility which said office deems sufficient to satisfy any claim. The office of emergency medical services shall establish by regulation satisfactory kinds of coverage and limits of insurance for each applicant of either licensure or certification, provided until such time as such regulations are promulgated the following shall be the required limits for licensure: (1) For damages by reason of personal injury to, or the death of, one person on account of any accident, of at least one hundred thousand dollars, and more than one person on account of any accident, of at least three hundred thousand dollars, (2) for damage to property of at least twenty-five thousand dollars and (3) for malpractice in the care of one passenger of at least one hundred thousand dollars, and for more than one passenger of at least three hundred thousand dollars. A certificate of such proof shall be filed with the office of emergency medical services. Upon determination by the office of emergency medical services that an applicant is financially responsible, properly certified and otherwise qualified to operate a commercial ambulance service, the office of emergency medical services shall issue a license effective for one year to such applicant. If the office of emergency services determines that an applicant for either a certificate or license is not so qualified, it shall notify such applicant of the denial of his application with a statement of the reasons for such denial. Such applicant shall have thirty days to request a hearing on the denial of said application.

(b) Any person or emergency medical services organization which does not maintain standards or violates regulations promulgated under any section of this act to which it is subject may have its license or certification suspended or revoked after notice by certified mail to such person or organization of the facts or conduct which warrant the intended action. Such emergency medical services organization shall have an opportunity to show compliance with all requirements for the retention of such certificate or license. In the conduct of any investigation by the office of emergency medical services of alleged violations of the standards or regulations promulgated under the provisions of this act, the director of such office may issue subpoenas requiring the attendance of witnesses and the production by any medical services organization or person of reports, records, tapes or other documents which concern the allegations under investigation.

(c) Any emergency medical service organization aggrieved by an act or decision of the office of emergency medical services regarding certification or licensure may appeal in the manner provided by chapter 54 of the general statutes, as amended.

(d) The office of emergency medical services shall issue a temporary ambulance or rescue operation permit to any service organization which submits satisfactory evidence to the office of emergency medical services that it was actively engaged in operating an ambulance or rescue service on January 1, 1974. Such temporary licenses shall expire one year from the date of issuance.

(e) Any person guilty of any of the following acts shall be fined not more than two hundred fifty dollars, or imprisoned not more than three months, or be both fined and imprisoned: (1) In any application to the office of emergency medical services or in any proceeding before it, or in any investigation made by it or on its authority, knowingly makes any false statement or representation, or, with knowledge of its falsity, files or causes to be filed with the office of emergency medical services any false statement or representation in a required application or statement; (2) issues, circulates or publishes, or causes to be issued, circulated or published any form of advertisement or circular for the purpose of soliciting business which contains any statement that is false or misleading, or otherwise likely to deceive a reader thereof, with knowledge that it contains such false, misleading or deceptive statement; (3) in any respect wilfully violates or fails to comply with any provision of this act or wilfully violates or fails, omits or neglects to obey or comply with any regulation, order, decision or license, or any part or provisions thereof; (4) with one or more other persons, conspires to violate any license or order issued by the office of emergency medical services or any provision of this act.

Sec. 10. (NEW) (a) Each ambulance or rescue vehicle used by an ambulance or rescue service shall be registered with the motor vehicle department pursuant to chapter 246 of the general statutes. Said motor vehicle department shall not issue a certificate of registration for any such ambulance or rescue vehicle unless the applicant for such certificate of registration presents to said department a safety certificate from the office of emergency services certifying that said ambulance or rescue vehicle has been inspected by said office and has met the minimum standards prescribed by the office and the commission. Each vehicle so registered with said department shall be inspected annually thereafter by said office on or before the anniversary date of the issuance of the certificate of registration. Each inspector, upon determining that such ambulance or rescue vehicle meets the standards of safety and equipment prescribed by said office, shall affix a safety certificate to such vehicle in such manner and form as said office shall designate, and such sticker shall be so placed as to be readily visible to any person in the rear compartment of such vehicle.

(b) The department of motor vehicles shall suspend or revoke the certificate of registration of any vehicle inspected under the provisions of this section upon certification from said office of emergency medical services that such ambulance or rescue vehicle has failed to meet the minimum standards prescribed by said office.

Sec. 11. (NEW) (a) The comprehensive health planning "b" agencies shall be the areawide planning and coordinating agencies for emergency medical services and shall provide continuous evaluation of emergency medical services for their respective geographic areas.

(b) Each comprehensive health planning "b" agency shall develop a plan for the delivery of emergency medical services in its area. Such plan shall include an evaluation of the current effectiveness of emergency medical services and detail the needs for the future, and shall contain specific goals for the delivery of emergency medical services within their respective geographic areas, a time frame for achievement of such goals, cost data for the development of such goals, and performance standards for the evaluation of such goals. Special emphasis in such plan shall be placed upon coordinating the existing services into a comprehensive system. Such plan shall contain provisions for, but shall not be limited to, the following: (1) Clearly defined geographic regions to be serviced by each provider including cooperative arrangements with other providers and backup services; (2) an adequate number of trained personnel for staffing of ambulances, communications facilities and hospital emergency rooms, with emphasis on former military personnel trained in allied health fields; (3) a communications system that includes a central dispatch center, two-way radio communication between the ambulance and the receiving hospital and a universal emergency telephone number and (4) a public education program that stresses the need for adequate training in basic life-saving techniques and cardio-pulmonary resuscitation. Such plan shall be submitted to the commission no later than December 31, 1974. The "b" agency shall perform its functions in cooperation with each appropriate emergency medical services council as established by section 12 of this act.

Sec. 12. (NEW) There shall be established an emergency medical service council in each region. Such regions shall correspond to the comprehensive health planning agency regions, provided if more than one emergency medical services council was in existence within such region on the effective date of this act, such councils shall continue in existence. Opportunity for membership shall be available to all appropriate representatives of emergency medical services including, but not limited to, one representative from each of the following: (a) Local governments, (b) fire and law enforcement officials, (c) medical and nursing professions, including mental health, paraprofessional and other allied health professionals; (d) providers of ambulance services, at least one of which shall be a member of a volunteer ambulance association, (e) institutions of higher education, (f) federal agencies involved in the delivery of health care, and (g) consumers. All emergency medical service councils including those in existence on the effective date of this act shall submit to the commission information concerning the organizational structure and council bylaws for commission approval. The commission shall foster the development of emergency medical service councils in each region.

Sec. 13. (NEW) Each emergency medical services council shall (1) review and within thirty days forward to the commission, together with its comments, the emergency medical services plan submitted by the "b" agency within its region, (2) advise the "b" agencies within its region on matters of policy and priority regarding emergency medical services and (3) in cooperation with the "b" agency within its region, review and within sixty days forward to the commission, together with its recommendations, all grant and contract applications for federal and state funds pertaining to emergency medical services from the following entities within its region: (a) A unit of local government, (B) a public entity administering a compact or other regional arrangement or consortium or (C) any other public entity or any nonprofit private agency.

Sec. 14. (NEW) There shall be a regional emergency medical services coordinator in each region who shall be appointed by the emergency medical services council or councils within the region subject to the approval of the respective "b" agencies and the commission. In those regions where no emergency medical services council exists such coordinator shall be appointed by the "b" agency with the approval of the commission.

Sec. 15. (NEW) The regional emergency medical services coordinator shall be responsible for: (1) Facilitating the work of the "b" agency and the council in developing the plan for the coordination of emergency medical services within the region, (2) implementation of the regional plan formulated by the regional "b" agency pursuant to subsection (b) of section 11 of this act, (3) continuous monitoring and evaluation of all emergency medical services in that region and (4) making a complete inventory of all personnel, facilities and equipment within the region related to the delivery of emergency medical services pursuant to guidelines established by the commission.

Sec. 16. (NEW) (a) All state agencies which are concerned with the emergency medical service delivery system shall, to the fullest extent consistent with their authorities under state law administered by them, carry out programs under their control in such a manner as to further the policy of establishing a coordinated statewide emergency medical service system.

(b) All such state agencies shall cooperate with the commission, the office of emergency medical services, and the regional "b" agencies, emergency medical service coordinators and emergency medical services councils in developing the state emergency medical services program under this act.

(c) All state agencies concerned with the statewide emergency medical services system shall cooperate with the appropriate agencies of the United States or of other states or interstate agencies with respect to the planning and coordination of emergency medical services.

Sec. 17. (NEW) The sum of two hundred and seventy-five thousand dollars is appropriated for the fiscal year ending June 30, 1975, to carry out the provisions of this act to be allocated as follows: (1) Fifty thousand dollars to the office of emergency medical services within the department of health, as established by section 6 of this act, for personnel, office equipment and supplies and (2) two hundred twenty-five thousand dollars to the commission on hospitals and health care for personnel, office equipment and supplies for implementation of the comprehensive emergency medical care system. Said sum is appropriated from the sum appropriated to the finance advisory committee, under section 1 of substitute house bill 5709 of the current session, for the reserve for legislation affecting agency budgets.

Sec. 18. Chapter 397 of the general statutes is repealed.

Sec. 19. This act shall take effect July 1, 1974.

Appendix 11B

The Connecticut Emergency Medical Services Act of 1975

PUBLIC ACT NO. 75-112
AN ACT CONCERNING THE TRANSFER OF ALL EMERGENCY MEDICAL SERVICE AUTHORITY FROM THE COMMISSION ON HOSPITALS AND HEALTH CARE TO THE DEPARTMENT OF HEALTH.

Be it enacted by the Senate and House of Representatives in General Assembly convened:

Section 1. Section 19-73u of the general statutes is repealed and the following is substituted in lieu thereof:

As used in this chapter, (a) "emergency medical service system" means a system which provides for the arrangement of personnel, facilities, and equipment for the efficient, effective and coordinated delivery of health care services under emergency conditions; (b) "comprehensive health planning agency" means any health planning agency created pursuant to section 246 (b) of title 42 of the United States Code, as amended, hereinafter referred to as the "b" agency; (c) "patient" means an injured, ill, crippled or physically handicapped person requiring assistance and transportation; (d) "ambulance" means a motor vehicle specifically designed to carry patients; (e) "ambulance service" means an organization which transports patients; [(f) "commission" means the commission on hospitals and health care created pursuant to section 19-73c; (g)] *(f)* "emergency medical technician" means an individual who has successfully completed the training requirements established by the [commis-

241

sion] COMMISSIONER OF HEALTH and has been certified by the state department of health; [(h)] *(g)* "ambulance driver" means a person whose primary function is driving an ambulance; [(i)] *(h)* "emergency medical technician instructor" means a person who is certified by the state department of health to teach courses, the completion of which are required in order to become an emergency medical technician; [(j)] *(i)* "communications facility" means any facility housing the personnel and equipment for handling the emergency communications needs of a particular geographic area; [(k)] *(j)* "life saving equipment" means equipment used by emergency medical personnel for the stabilization and treatment of patients; [(l)] *(k)* "emergency medical service organization" means any organization whether public, private or voluntary which offers transportation or treatment services to patients under emergency conditions; [(m)] *(l)* "invalid coach" means a vehicle used exclusively for the transportation of nonambulatory patients to or from either a medical facility or the patient's home in non-emergency situations or utilized in emergency situations as a back-up vehicle when insufficient emergency vehicles exist; [(n)] *(m)* "rescue service" means any organization, whether profit or nonprofit, whose primary purpose is to search for persons who have become lost or to render emergency service to persons who are in dangerous or perilous circumstances; [and (o)] *(n)* "provider" means any person, corporation or organization, whether profit or nonprofit, whose primary purpose is to deliver medical care or services, including such related medical care services as ambulance transportation; AND *(o)* "COMMISSIONER" MEANS THE COMMISSIONER OF HEALTH ACTING THROUGH THE OFFICE OF EMERGENCY MEDICAL SERVICES.

Sec. 2. Section 19-73v of the general statutes is repealed and the following is substituted in lieu thereof:

The [commission] STATE DEPARTMENT OF HEALTH shall be the state agency responsible for the planning, coordination and administration of a statewide emergency medical care service system. The [commission] COMMISSIONER OF HEALTH with the advice of the Connecticut advisory committee on emergency medical services, as established in section 19-73x, shall set policy and establish statewide priorities for emergency medical services utilizing the services of the state department of health and the "b" agencies and their associated emergency medical service councils, as established by section 19-73ee.

Sec. 3. Section 19-73w of the general statutes is repealed and the following is substituted in lieu thereof:

The [commission] COMMISSIONER shall: (a) With the advice of the Connecticut advisory committee on emergency medical services as established in section 19-73x, develop and annually update a statewide plan for the coordinated delivery of emergency medical services, which plan shall take into account the needs of the "b" agencies. The plan shall contain: (1) Specific goals for the delivery of such emergency medical services; (2) a time frame for achievement of such goals; (3) cost data and alternative funding sources for the development of such goals; and (4) performance standards for the evaluation of such goals;

(b) Annually inventory or cause to be inventoried emergency medical services resources within the state, including facilities, equipment, and personnel, for the purposes of determining the need for additional services and the effectiveness of existing services;

(c) Review and evaluate all areawide plans developed by the "b" agencies pursuant to section 19-73dd in order to insure conformity with standards issued by [the commission] SAID COMMISSIONER;

(d) Within thirty days of their receipt, review all grant and contract applications for federal or state funds concerning emergency medical services or related activities for conformity to policy guidelines and forward such application to the appropriate agency, when required;

(e) Establish such minimum standards and adopt such regulations in accordance with the provisions of chapter 54, as may be necessary to develop the following components of an emergency medical service system: (1) Communications, which shall include, but not be limited to, equipment, radio frequencies and operational procedures; (2) transportation services, which shall include, but not be limited to, vehicle type, design, condition and maintenance, life saving equipment and operational procedure; (3) training, which shall include, but not be limited to, emergency medical technicians, communications personnel, paraprofessionals associated with emergency medical services, firefighters and state and local police; (4) emergency medical service facilities, which shall include, but not be limited to, categorization of emergency departments as to their treatment capabilities and ancillary services;

(f) Coordinate training of all personnel related to emergency medical services;

(g) Develop or cause to be developed a data collection system which shall include a method of uniform patient record keeping which will follow a patient from initial entry into the emergency medical service system through discharge from the emergency room;

(h) Develop a program for public education and information which takes into account the needs of visitors to as well as residents of the state;

(i) Establish rates for the conveyance of patients in commercial ambulance vehicles and invalid coaches provided the present rates established by the public utilities commission for such vehicles shall remain in effect until such time as the [commission] COMMISSIONER establishes a new rate schedule as provided herein;

(j) No later than December 31, 1975, and annually thereafter submit a report to the governor and general assembly which shall include, but not be limited to, the following: (1) An accounting of all federal and state funds expended for emergency medical services in the state; (2) a statement and evaluation of the accomplishments of the office of [the statewide deputy director of] emergency medical services during the preceding year together with a description of goals for the upcoming year; and (3) recommendations for any legislation which [the commission] SAID COMMISSIONER feels will facilitate a complete coordinated emergency medical services system;

(k) If no "b" agency exists within a region, develop in conjunction with the regional coordinator, as established by section 19-73gg, an emergency medical services plan for such region, such plan to conform with the requirements of section 19-73dd.

Sec. 4. Subsection (a) of section 19-73x of the general statutes is repealed and the following is substituted in lieu thereof:

(a) There is established a Connecticut advisory committee on emergency medical services which shall advise the [commission] COMMISSIONER OF HEALTH regarding comprehensive emergency medical services. Said advisory committee shall be composed of twenty-five members appointed by the governor and shall include at least one representative each of the following: (1) Institutions of higher education; (2) police and fire officials; (3) hospital representatives; (4) federal agencies involved in health care; (5) medical, nursing and mental health officials; (6) provider representation, including one representative of volunteer ambulance associations; (7) third party payors; (8) paraprofessionals; (9) private nonprofit service agencies and (10) officials of state agencies which are concerned with the emergency medical service delivery system. ON OR BEFORE JULY 1, 1975, THE GOVERNOR SHALL APPOINT NINE MEMBERS FOR A TERM OF THREE YEARS, EIGHT MEMBERS FOR A TERM OF TWO YEARS AND EIGHT MEMBERS FOR A TERM OF ONE YEAR. THEREAFTER, ALL MEMBERS SHALL BE APPOINTED FOR TERMS OF THREE YEARS AND UNTIL THEIR SUCCESSORS ARE APPOINTED AND HAVE QUALIFIED.

Sec. 5. Section 19-73z of the general statutes is repealed and the following is substituted in lieu thereof:

There shall be established within the state department of health an office of emergency medical services. The office shall be responsible for (a) the licensure or certification of the following: (1) Ambulance operations, ambulance drivers, emergency medical technicians, and communications personnel; (2) emergency room facilities and communications facilities and (3) transportation equipment, including land, sea and air vehicles used for transportation of patients to emergency facilities [and]; (b) periodic inspections of life saving equipment, of emergency facilities and of emergency transportation vehicles to insure that state standards are maintained; and *(c)* PERFORM SUCH OTHER DUTIES AND FUNCTIONS AS ARE ASSIGNED TO SAID OFFICE BY THE COMMISSIONER OF HEALTH. [The office shall report its findings to the commission.]

Sec. 6. Subsection (a) of section 19-73aa of the general statutes is repealed and the following is substituted in lieu thereof:

(a) There shall be a director of the office of emergency medical services as established in section 19-73z who shall be appointed by and responsible to the commissioner of health. The director shall carry out the duties of the office of emergency medical services as provided in said section. [and] THE COMMISSIONER shall be responsible for adopting regulations concerning the methods and conditions for licensure and certification of the operations, facilities and equipment enumerated in said section and regulations regarding complaint procedures for the public and any emergency medical service organization. Such regulations shall be adopted in accordance with the provisions of chapter 54 and shall be in conformity with the policies and standards established by the [commission] COMMISSIONER. All regulations adopted by the ambulance commission and in force on June 30, 1974, shall remain in effect until such time as new regulations WHICH REPEAL, AMEND OR REPLACE SPECIFIC REGULATIONS concerning the methods and conditions for licensure and certification of the operations, facilities and equipment enumerated in said section and regulations regarding complaint procedures for the public and any emergency medical service organization are adopted by the [director of the office of emergency medical services] COMMISSIONER in accordance with the provisions of this section.

Sec. 7. Section 19-73bb of the general statutes is repealed and the following is substituted in lieu thereof:

(a) No person shall operate any ambulance service or rescue service without a certificate issued by the office of emergency medical services. No person shall operate a commercial ambulance or commercial rescue service without both a certificate and a license issued by the office of emergency medical services. A certificate shall be issued to any volunteer commercial or municipal ambulance service which shows proof satisfactory to the [commission] COMMISSIONER, of meeting the minimum standards of [the commission] SAID COMMISSIONER in the areas of training, equipment and personnel. Applicants for a license shall use the forms prescribed by the office of emergency medical services and shall submit such application to the office of emergency medical services accompanied by an annual fee of one hundred dollars. Each applicant for licensure OTHER THAN A VOLUNTEER AMBULANCE OR RESCUE SERVICE shall furnish proof of financial responsibility which said office deems sufficient to satisfy any claim. The [office of emergency medical services] COMMISSIONER OF HEALTH shall establish by regulation satisfactory kinds of coverage and limits of insurance for each applicant of either licensure or certification, provided until such time as such regulations are promulgated the following shall be the required limits for licensure: (1) For damages by reason of personal injury to, or the death of, one person on account of any accident, of at least one hundred thousand dollars, and more than one person on account of any accident, of at least three hundred thousand dollars, (2) for damage to property of at least twenty-five thousand dollars and (3) for malpractice in the care of one passenger of at least one hundred thousand dollars, and for more than one passenger of at least three hundred thousand dollars. A certificate of such proof shall be filed with the office of emergency medical services. Upon determination by the office of emergency medical services that an applicant is financially responsible, properly certified and otherwise qualified to operate a commercial ambulance service, the office of emergency medical services shall issue a license effective for one year to such applicant. If the office of emergency services determines that an applicant for either a certificate or license is not so qualified, it shall notify such applicant of the denial of his application with a statement of the reasons for such denial. Such applicant shall have thirty days to request a hearing on the denial of said application.

(b) Any person or emergency medical services organization which does not maintain standards or violates regulations promulgated under any section of this chapter to which it is subject may have its license or certification suspended or revoked after notice by certified mail to such person or organization of the facts or conduct which warrant the intended action. Such emergency medical services organization shall have an opportunity to show compliance with all requirements for the retention of such certificate or license. In the conduct of any investigation by the office of emergency medical services of alleged violations of the standards or regulations promulgated under the provisions of this chapter, the [director of such office] COMMISSIONER may issue subpoenas requiring the attendance of witnesses and the production by any medical services organization or person of reports, records, tapes or other documents which concern the allegations under investigation.

(c) Any emergency medical service organization aggrieved by an act or decision of the office of emergency medical services regarding certification or licensure may appeal in the manner provided by chapter 54.

(d) [The] ON OR BEFORE DECEMBER 31, 1975, THE office of emergency medical services shall issue a temporary ambulance or rescue operation permit to any service organization which submits satisfactory evidence to the office of emergency medical services that it was actively engaged in operating an ambulance or rescue service on January 1, 1974. Such temporary licenses shall expire one year from the date of issuance.

(e) Any person guilty of any of the following acts shall be fined not more than two hundred fifty dollars, or imprisoned not more than three months, or be both fined and imprisoned: (1) In any application to the office of emergency medical services or in any proceeding before it, or in any investigation made by it or on its authority, knowingly makes any false statement or representation, or, with knowledge of its falsity, files or causes to be filed with the office of emergency medical services any false statement or representation in a required application or statement; (2) issues, circulates or publishes, or causes to be issued, circulated or published any form of advertisement or circular for the purpose of soliciting business which contains any statement that is false or misleading, or otherwise likely to deceive a reader thereof, with knowledge that it contains such false, misleading or deceptive statement; (3) in any respect wilfully violates or fails to comply with any provision of this chapter or wilfully violates or fails, omits or neglects to obey or comply with any regulation, order, decision or license, or any part or provisions thereof; (4) with one or more other persons, conspires to violate any license or order issued by the office of emergency medical services or any provision of this chapter.

Sec. 8. Section 19-73cc of the general statutes is repealed and the following is substituted in lieu thereof:

(a) Each ambulance or rescue vehicle used by an ambulance or rescue service shall be registered with the motor vehicle department pursuant to chapter 246. Said motor vehicle department shall not issue a certificate of registration for any such ambulance or rescue vehicle unless the applicant for such certificate of registration presents to said department a safety certificate from the office of emergency services certifying that said ambulance or rescue vehicle has been inspected by said office and has met the minimum standards prescribed by the [office and the commission] COMMISSIONER. Each vehicle so registered with said department shall be inspected annually thereafter by said office on or before the anniversary date of the issuance of the certificate of registration. Each inspector, upon determining that such ambulance or rescue vehicle meets the standards of safety and equipment prescribed by said office, shall affix a safety certificate to such vehicle in such manner and form as said office shall designate, and such sticker shall be so placed as to be readily visible to any person in the rear compartment of such vehicle.

(b) The department of motor vehicles shall suspend or revoke the certificate of registration of any vehicle inspected under the provisions of this section upon certification from said office of emergency medical services that such ambulance or rescue vehicle has failed to meet the minimum standards prescribed by said [office] COMMISSIONER.

Sec. 9. Subsection (b) of section 19-73dd of the general statutes is repealed and the following is substituted in lieu thereof:

(b) Each comprehensive health planning "b" agency shall develop a plan for the delivery of emergency medical services in its area. Such plan shall include an evaluation of the current effectiveness of emergency medical services and detail the needs for the future, and shall contain specific goals for the delivery of emergency medical services within their respective geographic areas, a time frame for achievement of such goals, cost data for the development of such goals, and performance standards for the evaluation of such goals. Special emphasis in such plan shall be placed upon coordinating the existing services into a comprehensive system. Such plan shall contain provisions for, but shall not be limited to, the following: (1) Clearly defined geographic regions to be serviced by each provider including cooperative arrangements with other providers and backup services; (2) an adequate number of trained personnel for staffing of ambulances, communications facilities and hospital emergency rooms, with emphasis on former military personnel trained in allied health fields; (3) a communications system that includes a central dispatch center, two-way radio communication between the ambulance and the receiving hospital and a universal emergency telephone number and (4) a public education program that stresses the need for adequate training in basic life-saving techniques and cardio-pulmonary resuscitation. Such plan shall be submitted to the [commission] COMMISSIONER OF HEALTH no later than December 31, 1974. The "b" agency shall perform its functions in cooperation with each appropriate emergency medical services council as established by section 19-73ee.

Sec. 10. Section 19-73ee of the general statutes is repealed and the following is substituted in lieu thereof:

There shall be established an emergency medical service council in each region. Such regions shall correspond to the comprehensive health planning agency regions, provided if more than one emergency medical services council was in existence within such region on July 1, 1974, such councils shall continue in existence. Opportunity for membership shall be available to all appropriate representatives of emergency medical services including, but not limited to, one representative from each of the following: (a) Local governments, (b) fire and law enforcement officials, (c) medical and nursing professions, including mental health, paraprofessional and other allied health professionals, (d) providers of ambulance services, at least one of which shall be a member of a volunteer ambulance association, (e) institutions of higher education, (f) federal agencies involved in the delivery of health care, and (g) consumers. All emergency medical service councils including those in existence on July 1, 1974, shall submit to the [commission] COMMISSIONER OF HEALTH information concerning the organizational structure and council bylaws for [commission] HIS approval. The [commission] COMMISSIONER shall foster the development of emergency medical service councils in each region.

Sec. 11. Section 19-73ff of the general statutes is repealed and the following is substituted in lieu thereof:

Each emergency medical services council shall (1) review and within thirty days forward to the [commission] COMMISSIONER OF HEALTH, together with its comments, the emergency medical services plan submitted by the "b" agency within its region, (2) advise the "b" agencies within its region on matters of policy and priority regarding emergency medical services and (3) in cooperation with the "b" agency within its region, review and within sixty days forward to the [commission] COMMISSIONER, together with its recommendations, all grant and contract applications for federal and state funds pertaining to emergency medical services from the following entities within its region: (A) A unit of local government, (B) a public entity administering a compact or other regional arrangement or consortium or (C) any other public entity or any nonprofit private agency.

Sec. 12. Section 19-73gg of the general statutes is repealed and the following is substituted in lieu thereof:

There shall be a regional emergency medical services coordinator in each region who shall be appointed by the emergency medical services council or councils within the region subject to the approval of the respective "b" agencies and the [commission] COMMIS-SIONER. In those regions where no emergency medical services council exists such coordinator shall be appointed by the "b" agency with the approval of [the commission] SAID COMMISSIONER.

Sec. 13. Section 19-73hh of the general statutes is repealed and the following is substituted in lieu thereof:

The regional emergency medical services coordinator shall be responsible for: (1) Facilitating the work of the "b" agency and the council in developing the plan for the coordination of emergency medical services within the region, (2) implementation of the regional plan formulated by the regional "b" agency pursuant to subsection (b) of section 19-73dd, (3) continuous monitoring and evaluation of all emergency medical services in that region and (4) making a complete inventory of all personnel, facilities and equipment within the region related to the delivery of emergency medical services pursuant to guidelines established by the [commission] COMMISSIONER OF HEALTH.

Sec. 14. Subsection (b) of section 19-73ii of the general statutes is repealed and the following is substituted in lieu thereof:

(b) All such state agencies shall cooperate with [the commission,] the office of emergency medical services, and the regional "b" agencies, emergency medical service coordinators and emergency medical services councils in developing the state emergency medical services program under this chapter.

Sec. 15. (NEW) All existing staff, equipment and office supplies and all budgeted funds for the emergency medical services division of the commission on hospitals and health care are hereby transferred to and made part of the office of emergency medical services.

Sec. 16. Section 19-73y of the general statutes is repealed.

Sec. 17. (NEW) The balance of 1974–1975 unencumbered appropriation to the commission on hospitals and health care for emergency medical services are transferred to the state department of health for the purposes of this act.

Sec. 18. This act shall take effect from its passage.

Appendix 11C

Regulations for Emergency Medical Services—Connecticut State Department of Health (1975)

Rules and Regulations

CHAPTER I

In accordance with the provisions of Section 4-168 of the Connecticut General Statutes, as amended, the Commissioner of Health hereby adopts the following regulations under authority of Public Act 75-112.

NEW
19-73w-1—Administration
A. *The Commissioner of Health (hereafter referred to as the Commissioner)* is charged in P.A. 75-112, Sections 2 and 3, with the development and coordination of a statewide Emergency Medical Services System. Further, the *Commissioner* is charged to utilize the services of the "b" agencies in the development of the system. Therefore, each Comprehensive Health Planning "b" agency or a comparable agency acceptable to the *Commissioner* shall provide regional EMS planning services as specified in 19-73w(a)-(k) and these regulations, Chapter I, 19-73w-1 to 5. These planning services will be in conformance with the EMS Act of *1975* and these regulations and in a form and substance suitable to the *Commissioner*.

B.   A region shall be composed of the towns so designated by the *Commissioner* and comprising the Regional EMS Planning Agency. Variations from this configuration for Emergency Medical Service planning may be approved by the *Commissioner* where it can be demonstrated to be necessary for effective regional planning and coordination and such changes are agreeable to the agencies and towns.

19-73w-2—Regional Coordinator

A.   Each regional Emergency Medical Services planning agency functioning pursuant to Section 19-73w-1 of this chapter shall employ a "Regional Coordinator" as specified in 19-73gg, G.S. and this section of *Connecticut State Department of Health* regulations.

B.   The duties of the Regional Coordinator shall be limited to Emergency Medical Services.

C.   The Regional Coordinator shall be responsible for the following services:

1.   Make a complete inventory of all personnel, facilities and equipment related to the delivery of emergency medical services within that region.

2.   Facilitate the work of the Regional EMS Planning Agency and Regional EMS Council in developing the regional Emergency Medical Service plan.

3.   Implement the regional EMS plan through such activities as establishing mutual aid and response plans between communities in the region.

4.   Continuously monitor and evaluate all emergency medical services in that region.

5.   Maintain liaison with the Director OEMS as to all developments in EMS policy.

6.   Serve as liaison between the Regional EMS Planning Agency and the Regional EMS Council.

7.   Act as staff for the Regional Emergency Medical Service Council.

8.   Coordinate Emergency Medical Service activity relating to disaster planning.

9.   Assist in establishing mutual aid and response plans.

D.   The Regional Coordinator should have the following qualifications and background:

1.   Skills in administration oriented towards program management.

2. Knowledge of Emergency Medical Service allowing him to relate to various Emergency Medical Service personnel.
3. Knowledge of transport, communications and lifesaving equipment utilized within the Emergency Medical Service system.
4. Knowledge of data gathering and analysis techniques.
5. Experience of working with or within community organizational structures.
6. An educational background or experience in the above areas.

19-73w-3—Regional Emergency Medical Services Councils

A. In each region there shall be established an Emergency Medical Services advisory council to provide advice and guidance on policy to the Emergency Medical Services planning agency and the regional coordinator(s) as to the region's problems, needs and priorities in the area of Emergency Medical Services.

B. The council members shall be active participants in formulating the region's Emergency Medical Services plan as developed by the planning agency. The planning agency shall submit the plan to the council which shall have 30 days to forward the plan along with comments to the Commissioner.

C. The structure of the council and its by-laws shall be submitted to the Commissioner for review and approval. The opportunity for membership and active participation shall be available but not limited to all providers, professionals, or agencies substantially affected by actions of the council. Care should be taken to provide equitable geographic representation for the entire region and a balance of categories so that control does not reside in one town or one interested group. The following entities, among others, should be represented:
1. Local government
2. Fire and law enforcement
3. Medical, nursing, allied health professionals
4. Providers of ambulance service including at least one volunteer ambulance service if appropriate for the region
5. Emergency treatment facility personnel
6. Consumers, including minority groups, if appropriate for the region
7. Planning agencies.

C. The regional Emergency Medical Services coordinator shall provide necessary staff assistance for the council.

D. Any changes in the officers of the council shall be reported to the Director OEMS within 30 days. The complete membership of the council shall be submitted annually.

E. If any substantial changes in council structure or organization are undertaken, approval pursuant to19-73w-3B shall be sought.

F. The council shall assist the regional Emergency Medical Service planning agency with review and comment on all grant applications for federal or state funds, provided such funds are related to the delivery of Emergency Medical Services and that the applications affect all or part of the region.

19-73w-4—Regional Emergency Medical Services Inventory

A. An inventory of all Emergency Medical Service resources in each region of the state as defined in 19-73w-1B shall be made or updated annually. The designated regional Emergency Medical Service planning agency shall prepare for submission to the Commissioner by September 30 of each year, in a form and manner acceptable to the Commissioner, a detailed description of current Emergency Medical Service resources including current geographic areas of responsibility of all key elements of the Emergency Medical Service System. The inventory shall be made in conformance with planning outlines for Emergency Medical Services recommended by the Departments of Transportation, Health, Education and Welfare. All elements must be currently inventoried and drawn from reports less than three months old.

B. The inventory shall furnish data under the following categories:

1. *Ambulance services*—number, type (i.e. volunteer, commercial), location, usage, method of dispatch, financial status, etc.

2. *Vehicles and equipment*—numbers and types of ambulances, chair cars and rescue vehicles, age, equipment carried, etc.

3. *Personnel*—numbers of personnel by agency affiliation (i.e. physician, nurse, Emergency Medical Technician-Ambulance, American Red Cross advanced, etc.) and time commitment (i.e. full time, part time, on call, etc.).

4. *Training*—location and frequency of training, number of people trained, physicians, nurse, EMT-A, ARC advanced, dispatcher, in-service, seminars (include specific skills).

5. *Facilities*—emergency departments by area distribution, size, usage, staffing patterns, category, services available, and special facilities (i.e. CIU, CCU, Burn unit, etc.).

6. *Communications*—method of access, dispatch, medical consultation, radio frequencies used, location of dispatch centers, interface with other dispatch centers, staffing patterns, units which are on network, etc.
7. *Consumer education*—How are people currently told about availability of Emergency Medical Services, training programs, Emergency Medical Services planning.
8. *Evaluation*—How is current Emergency Medical Service capability monitored? How is patient outcome evaluated. What permanent records are maintained by various system elements.
9. *Patient flow pattern*—give a description of current, typical patient flow patterns for an emergency situation.
10. *Disaster plan*—current plan for dealing with multi-casualty situations, including as much detail as possible.
11. *Mutual aid and response plans*—What is current mutual aid and response arrangement, if any, and to what extent is it formalized (i.e. oral, written, not specified).
12. Detailed demographic information
    a. *Population*—by age, sex, area distribution
    b. *Population densities*—by cities and planning areas. Estimate the number of people residing in areas of more than 50,000 population.
    c. *Medical personnel*—Emergency room doctors, nurses, allied health personnel and ambulance personnel by area distribution.
13. *Detailed area characteristics*—Maps and charts should be used to graphically describe the area covered by the inventory.
    a. Roads (state and federal mileage)
    b. High accident locations on major roads
    c. Geographic conditions
    d. Climatological conditions as they affect ground and air transport
    e. Economic and social conditions of the population
    f. Epidemiological characteristics
    g. Other factors—industrial complexes, occupational dominance, related hazards, etc.

19-73w-5—Regional Emergency Medical Services Plan
A. There shall be developed for each region (defined in 19-73w-1 B) of the state a plan for implementing an Emergency Medical Services System. The initial plan shall be completed by December

31 and revised and refiled annually on the same date. The plan which shall be submitted to the Commissioner by the region shall be in a form and content acceptable to the Commissioner. The plan shall include, but not be limited to, elements B through P of this section with the following details for each:

1. An evaluation of current needs and effectiveness
2. Specific goals for meeting future needs
3. Specific time frame during which each goal shall be achieved
4. Cost data for the achievement of each goal
5. Methodology which shall be used to evaluate the achievement of each goal.

B. The plan shall provide adequate numbers of trained personnel:
1. Detailed training levels of all involved personnel, including but not limited to, Emergency Room physicians, Emergency Room nurses, allied health professionals, ambulance drivers and attendants, fire rescue, police, communications personnel, instructors in above areas.
2. Detailed staffing patterns for all EMS system elements.
3. Detailed method of ensuring that all EMS system elements are assured of adequate staffing on a 24-hour basis.

C. Provides adequate and continuous training for EMS personnel:
1. Detailed initial training programs for all personnel, i.e. ARC, EMT-A, CIM, EMT-II, physicians, nurses, etc.
2. Detailed in-service training for Emergency room personnel, ambulance and fire, police, etc.

D. Provides central communications for an EMS System:
1. Utilizes screening for system entry
2. Utilizes a central access number, preferably 911
3. Provides direct communications between all providers.

E. Provides adequate vehicles, ground, air and water
1. Meet requirements for: locations, design, performance and equipment
2. Provides training for operators.

F. Provides adequate Emergency room facilities which are categorized.

G. Provides access and transportation to critical care and specialty units.

H. Provides for effective utilization of each public safety agency providing emergency service in the region.

I. Provides for public input into policy decisions.

J. Provides EMS without inquiry into ability to pay.

K. Provides for emergency transfer.

L. Provides record-keeping system which originates with entry into system and end with discharge from emergency department.

M. Provide public information which:
1. Provides visitors as well as residents with information as to methods of access into system
2. Provides information as to availability of first-aid training in region
3. Encourages obtaining of first-aid training by general public.

N. Provides for periodic review of EMS system.

O. Provides a detailed disaster plan.

P. Provides a mutual aid and response plan in writing for all elements of the EMS system.

19-73w-6 through 299 reserved.

CHAPTER II—OPERATIONAL STANDARDS AND PROCEDURES FOR EMS

19-73w-300—Definitions
For the purposes of this chapter, the definitions in 19-73u, G.S. and the definitions used in Section 19-73w-400 shall apply.

A. Persons who file applications for license or certification for ambulance operations and other EMS operations and rescue services shall be defined as Providers under these regulations.

19-73w-301—Powers and duties of the Connecticut
State Department of Health
The Connecticut State Department of Health is the state agency responsible for the planning, coordination, and administration of a statewide emergency medical care service system. The Connecticut State Department of Health through the Commissioner shall with the advice of the CAC/EMS set policy and establish statewide priorities for emergency medical services; and establish such minimum standards and adopt such regulations in accordance with the provisions of Chapter 54 of the General Statutes, as may be necessary to develop the components of an emergency medical service system as provided in 19-73w, G.S.

19-73w-302—Records
A. Each licensed or certified ambulance service shall maintain records of employees or members, training courses taken by employees or members, motor vehicle maintenance and a log of

each trip in a form and manner approved by the Commissioner. All of said records shall be maintained for inspection by a designated agency of the State of Connecticut upon reasonable notice to certified services and at any reasonable time without notice by entering the premises of licensed ambulance services.

B. Licensed ambulance services shall maintain business records at their business location. Such records shall be open for inspection by the licensing agency. The stock transfer books of corporations shall be considered part of such records for corporations.

19-73w-303 Reserved

19-73w-304—License Not Required
No license or certificate shall be required, under the provisions of 19-73w of the G.S. and Connecticut State Department of Health regulations, for a person operating an ambulance service, and no license shall be required under the provisions of P.A. 75-112 and Connecticut State Department of Health regulations for an ambulance driver and technician for such ambulance service, when such ambulance service is operated from a location or headquarters outside the state and transports patients from locations outside the state to locations within the state, or transports patients from locations within the state to locations outside the state; provided no such ambulance service shall be granted a primary service area in the state.

19-73w-305—Accident Reports
Each ambulance service shall report to the Office of Emergency Medical Services in the Connecticut State Department of Health any accident resulting in personal injury or property damage which was or may have been connected with or due to the operation of its property, as soon as may be reasonably possible after the occurrence of such accident but in no case later than five days after the accident. If such notice is given otherwise than in writing, it shall be confirmed by the filing of a written notice within five days after the occurrence of such accident.

19-73w-306—Ownership
Where patient care is shown to be adversely affected, persons employed by or holding elective or appointed office with a local unit of municipal town government may not own an interest in nor have a supervisory position with any commercial emergency ambulance firm providing service to such area under the jurisdiction of such local municipal town government.

19-73w-307—Advertising

Ambulance services shall not advertise emergency medical services or emergency personnel for any political subdivision which has designated a phone number to be used to obtain EMS. On or before April 15, 1976, each regional EMS council shall, in consultation with each political subdivision located within its jurisdictional area, designate a telephone number for EMS system access. The only EMS telephone numbers that may be placed in telephone directories will be the numbers designated by each regional EMS council and on file with OEMS. In the event any regional EMS council fails to designate an EMS access number as provided herein, OEMS shall, in consultation with each political subdivision affected, designate such a telephone number. It is not the intent of this regulation to interfere with the normal publicity used by volunteer ambulances to raise funds and recruit personnel.

19-73w-308—Records

All data collected from the promulgation of these regulations shall be available to the Advisory Committee upon request.

CHAPTER III

These regulations shall establish minimum standards for the configuration and operation of an emergency medical service response system which shall cover every section of the State of Connecticut. While it is anticipated that most, if not all, EMS providers will substantially exceed these requirements, the citizenry of this state may expect *at least* this level of care if injured or ill.

19-73w-400—Definitions

All definitions used herein shall be those provided in P.A. 75-112 and the following:

A. *Service*—an activity specifically arranged to provide emergency medical services.

B. *Response Service*—a service specifically arranged to provide the ability to physically move from one location to another as a direct result of instructions or protocols established pursuant to providing emergency medical services.

C. *Designated Response Service*—a response service which has been assigned a primary service area for a specific category (R1-R5) of EMS responsibility and which has satisfactorily completed all necessary certification and licensure requirements.

D.　*PSA*—Primary Service Area—a specified geographic area within which there shall be one designated response service assigned as the first call service for a given category (R1-R5) of EMS response.

E.　*Council*—regional EMS council.

F.　*OEMS*—State of Connecticut, Department of Health, Office of Emergency Medical Services.

G.　*ARC*—American Red Cross.

H.　*AHA*—American Heart Association.

I.　*MRT*—Medical Response Technician.

J.　*EMT*—Emergency Medical Technician-Ambulance.

K.　*EMT-II*—Emergency Medical Technician-Advanced.

L.　*Crew Member*—a specifically assigned person to fulfill minimum regulation requirements.

M.　*At the Scene*—the immediate proximity of a location where a person requiring emergency medical assistance is situated.

N.　*CIM*—Federal Department of Transportation approved crash injury management program.

O.　*New Motor Vehicle*—means a motor vehicle, the equitable or legal title to which has never been transferred by a manufacturer, distributor or dealer to an ultimate consumer. *Ultimate consumer* means, with respect to a motor vehicle, the first person, other than a dealer, who, in good faith, purchases such motor vehicle for purposes other than resale.

P.　*Suitable Substitute*—an item, procedure or protocol determined appropriate by regional council and approved by the Commissioner.

Q.　*Paraprofessional Training Program*—ARC advanced first aid and emergency care, CIM, EMT-A, EMT-II.

19-73w-401—Categorization of Response Services

In order to develop a systems approach to the delivery of EMS, certain standard elements must be indicated. This section defines system elements by capability in order to provide sufficient flexibility to meet local needs while maintaining a minimum level of standards.

A.　R1—a designated response service which has the capability of providing the following at the scene of each EMS call to which it has responded: (While there is no requirement that any community designate an R1 responder, in communities where the average R2 response time is over ten minutes, it is highly recommended that an R1 be designated.)

As of 1/1/77

1.　A minimum of one certified medical response technician

    a. Bandaging material and dressings sufficient to control hemorrhage including venous and/or arterial hemorrhage.

    b. Oropharyngeal and/or mouth-to-mouth airways in infant, child and adult sizes. Such airways should be non-rigid, non-metal in construction.

    c. Poison treatment kit.

As of 6/1/80

    d. Two-way radio communications equipment compatible with EMS communications for the region/regions within which they operate:

2. The ability to perform at least the following:

    a. Respond to a call for EMS

    b. Control hemorrhage including arterial and/or venous hemorrhage

    c. Cardio-pulmonary resuscitation

    d. Dilute poison and/or induce vomiting

    e. Shock prevention, management

    f. Deliver a baby

    g. Perform triage

    h. Scene management

    i. Protect skeletal injuries.

B. R2—a designated response service which has the capability of providing at least the following at the scene of each EMS call to which it has responded:

1. A minimum of a *two-member crew* consisting of:

As of Effective Date of These Regulations

    a. *commercial licensed service*—two licensed EMT's, one of whom shall be in patient compartment attending the patient during all periods in which a patient is being transported. Effective on passage. All other crew members shall hold current certification in ARC advanced first aid (old course—27 hours) and an AHA CPR course or a suitable substitute as determined by the Commissioner.

As of 6/1/76

    b. *volunteer and municipal services*—One certified EMT who shall be in patient compartment attending the patient during all periods in which a patient is being transported and all other crew members shall hold current certification in ARC advanced first aid (old course—27 hours) and an AHA CPR course or a suitable substitute as determined by the Commissioner.

As of 6/1/77

    c. *volunteer and municipal services*—at least one certified EMT who shall be in patient compartment attending the patient during all periods in which a patient is being transported and one certified MRT.

As of 1/1/80

    d. All services shall be staffed by two certified EMT's, one of whom shall be in the patient compartment attending the patient during all periods in which a patient is being transported.

2. The ability to perform at least the following:
   a. Respond to a call for EMS
   b. Control hemorrhage including arterial and/or venous hemorrhage
   c. Perform cardio-pulmonary resuscitation
   d. Dilute poison and/or induce vomiting
   e. Shock prevention, management
   f. Deliver a baby
   g. Perform triage
   h. Scene management
   i. Immobilize and protect skeletal injuries
   j. Dress and protect burns
   k. Determine and relay vital signs
   l. Assess, manage and protect victims of medical emergencies
   m. Assess, manage and protect alcohol, drug and emotionally disturbed patients
   n. Provide transport to appropriate medical facilities
   o. Advanced life support techniques shall only be performed by R2 services when the decision to activate such techniques has been approved by the regional EMS council with the approval of the Commissioner. Specific protocols shall be developed by the physician component of regional council.

3. A *vehicle* which meets the following design criteria:
As of 1/1/77
   a. An especially designed patient transport vehicle with:
      (1) minimum 51″ head room in patient compartment measured from floor aisle space to head liner
      (2) minimum 114″ interior length in patient compartment from inside back door to rear of driver's compartment

(3) minimum 12″ unobstructed aisle space between primary patient stretcher and any obstruction for full length of primary patient stretcher on one side

(4) ability to achieve and maintain an average patient compartment temperature of 75° regardless of weather conditions

(5) electrical intercom or signal lights or an open partition to permit exchange of patient condition information between patient compartment and driver

(6) sufficient secure storage to permit secure loading and confinement of all items which could move freely about patient area in the event of a collision or roll over

(7) rotating or flashing warning lights visible 360° about vehicle

(8) mechanical and/or electronic siren

(9) two-way communications equipment compatible with the radio communications system for the region(s) in which such vehicle operates

(10) exterior identification visible 360° about vehicle identifying vehicle as an ambulance

(11) exterior identification visible on two opposing sides of vehicle identifying service vehicle is operated by.

As of 7/1/76

    b. Any new R2 vehicle being licensed as an ambulance shall meet or exceed the design criteria of General Services Administration specifications KKK-A-1822 dated January 2, 1974, as amended. Copies of current specifications are available upon request from OEMS.

As of 1/1/84

    c. Any vehicle licensed as an R2 vehicle in the state of Connecticut shall meet or exceed the design criteria of General Services Administration specifications KKK-A-1822 dated January 2, 1974, as amended. Copies of current specifications are available upon request from OEMS.

As of 7/1/76

4. Equipment as follows:

    a. All equipment shall be in working order and each crew member shall be thoroughly knowledgeable in its operation.

(1) Oxygen administration apparatus with 2 hours' supply at 7 lpm flow rate, regulator controlled flow rate permitting adjustment from a minimum of 2 lpm–10 lpm with visual indication of flow rate. Adaptors so that a minimum of 2 patients may be provided O_2 at the same time. A minimum of 2 each, bi-nasal cannulas and mouth/nose masks.

(2) Portable oxygen administration apparatus with 30 minutes' supply at 7 lpm flow rate, which is operable totally disattached from parent vehicle. Such unit shall be capable of accepting attachment to a bi-nasal cannula, mouth/nose mask or as enrichment feed to a forced ventilation unit.

(3) Suction apparatus capable of drawing a vacuum of 300 mm of mercury. Such unit shall be operable completely independent of parent vehicle for a minimum period of 15 minutes. Such suction apparatus shall be compatible with both rigid and flexible catheters and a minimum of 1 catheter and 1 spare shall be carried.

(4) Mechanical forced resuscitation unit. Such unit shall be either hand-operated (bag mask) or cycled only by operator manual control. (*Pressure cycled units are not acceptable.*) Such units shall be compatible with O_2 apparatus carried in the subject vehicle for purposes of oxygen enrichment. Such unit shall be compatible with infant, child and adult masks which shall be made of transparent material and shall be carried.

(5) Artificial airways—either mouth-to-mouth, oropharyngeal or other acceptable artificial airway maintenance devices in infant, child and adult sizes. A minimum of 1 and 1 spare for each size.

(6) Either commercial bite stick or some suitable substitute for maintaining an open-jawed position on an unconscious patient.

(7) Large dressings of the ABD or Multi-Trauma type. A minimum of six such dressings or a suitable substitute.

(8) Assorted dressings and bandages to permit hemorrhage control by direct pressure bandage on any area of the human body regardless of severity of hemorrhage.

(9) Aluminum foil, sterile vaseline gauze or other air excluding dressing material to permit air-tight seal of wounds to the chest cavity.

(10) Two sterile sheets or suitable substitute for isolating burn patients from exterior sources of contamination.

(11) Hare traction, Thomas half-ring or other suitable substitute for providing prolonged traction to a lower limb on a child or adult.

(12) Splinting material to permit immobilization and protection to any aspect of a child or adult limb in any position. A minimum of 1 spare shall be carried for each size of splint.

(13) Short back board with 2 straps minimum of 9' by 2", 3 cervical immobilization collars of assorted sizes (extrication type collars are recommended), forehead and chin restraints or other suitable substitute to permit the immobilization of suspected cervical fracture of a child or adult patient during removal from a confined space while in a seated position and during transport.

(14) A long wooden spine board with 2 - 9" straps or other suitable substitute to permit the immobilization and transport of a spinal column fracture without vertical or horizontal expansion, contraction or twisting. (A scoop type stretcher is not a suitable substitute for this item.)

(15) Commercial stair chair or other suitable substitute to permit the movement of a patient either up or down within a confined stairway.

(16) Blood pressure manometer, cuff and stethoscope or other suitable substitute for determining patient blood pressure both outside and inside of vehicle.

(17) Restraint devices of sufficient strength to restrain a violent adult and sufficiently padded to prevent chafing and/or injury to patient.

(18) A poison treatment kit consisting of a minimum of 2 oz. each of activated charcoal and syrup of Ipecac or some suitable substitute for each in addition to one-half gallon potable water.

(19) An obstetrical kit containing a minimum of 1 pair sterile gloves, scissors, umbilical cord clamps or tapes, sterile vaginal dressings, 2 towels, large plas-

tic bag, and swaddling material. (Aluminum foil is acceptable as swaddling material as are burn sheets.)

(20)   One emesis basin, 1 bed pan, and 1 urinal or suitable substitute.

(21)   Not less than 2 pillows and 2 sets of linen to include 2 sheets and 1 blanket per set.

(22)   A minimum of 2 10BC UL fire extinguishers, 1 carried in driver compartment and 1 in patient compartment.

(23)   At least two battery operated, hand-carried portable lights.

(24)   One wrecking bar minimum 24″ in length.

(25)   At least one multi-level cot with 2 patient securing straps. Such cot shall be removable from the ambulance, and provision shall be made for positive locking when the cot is positioned in the vehicle.

(26)   Glucose in a form easily ingested orally.

(27)   A paper bag or similar rebreathing device for use in treating hyperventilation syndrome.

(28)   A minimum of 3 hours' duration red-burning flares.

(29)   Two sets of sandbags.

C.   R5—a designated response service which has the capability of providing the following at the scene of each EMS call to which it has responded:

1.   A *crew* consisting of a minimum of two people who meet the following criteria:

As of 1/1/76

a.   One certified EMT-II, all other crew members certified EMT's

As of 1/1/77

b.   Two certified EMT-II's

c.   Or other suitable substitute

2.   The ability to perform at least the following:

a.   Respond to a call for EMS

b.   Control hemorrhage including arterial and/or venous hemorrhage

c.   Cardio-pulmonary resuscitation

d.   Dilute poison and/or induce vomiting

e.   Shock prevention, management

f.   Deliver a baby

g. Perform triage
h. Scene management
i. Immobilize and protect skeletal injuries
j. Dress and protect burns
k. Determine and relay vital signs
l. Assess, manage and protect victims of medical emergencies
m. Assess, manage and protect alcohol, drug and emotionally disturbed patients
n. Assess need for, initiate and maintain administration of IV fluids
o. Assess need for, initiate administration of selected medication both IV and IM
p. Defibrillate as needed
q. Transmit bio-medical information, to include EKG, from scene to supervising physician via two-way radio communication
r. Decision to activate n, o, p, q above shall be made by regional council with approval of Commissioner. Specific protocols for performance shall be developed by physician component of regional council.

3. The following equipment:
    a. Portable oxygen administration apparatus with 30 minutes' supply at 7 lpm flow rate, which is operable totally disattached from parent vehicle. Such unit shall be capable of accepting attachment to a bi-nasal cannula, mouth/nose mask or as enrichment feed to a forced ventilation unit.
    b. Suction apparatus capable of drawing a vacuum of 300 mm of mercury. Such unit shall be operable completely independent of parent vehicle for a minimum period of 15 minutes. Such suction apparatus shall be compatible with both rigid and flexible catheters and a minimum of 1 catheter and 1 spare shall be carried.
    c. Mechanical forced resuscitation unit. Such unit shall be either hand-operated (bag mask) or cycled only by operator manual control. (*Pressure cycled units are not acceptable.*) Such units shall be compatible with O_2 apparatus carried for purposes of oxygen enrichment. Such unit shall be compatible with infant, child and adult masks which shall be made of a transparent material and shall be carried.

d. Artificial airways—either mouth-to-mouth, oropharyngeal or other acceptable artificial airway maintenance devices in infant, child and adult sizes. A minimum of 1 and 1 spare for each size.

e. Either commercial bite stick or some other suitable substitute for maintaining an open-jawed position on an unconscious patient.

f. Large dressings of the ABD or Multi-Trauma type. A minimum of six such dressings or a suitable substitute.

g. Assorted dressings and bandages to permit hemorrhage control by direct pressure bandage on any area of the human body regardless of severity of hemorrhage.

h. Aluminum foil, sterile vaseline gauze or other air excluding dressing material to permit air-tight seal of wounds to the chest cavity.

i. Two sterile sheets or suitable substitute for isolating burn patients from exterior sources of contamination.

j. Hare traction, Thomas half-ring or other suitable substitute for providing prolonged traction to a lower limb on a child and/or adult.

k. Suitable splinting material to permit immobilization and protection to any aspect of a child or adult limb in any position. A minimum of 1 spare should be carried for each size of splint.

l. Short back board with 2 straps minimum 9′ × 2″, three cervical immobilization collars of assorted sizes (extrication type collars are recommended), forehead and chin restraints or other suitable substitute to permit the immobilization of a suspected cervical fracture of a child or adult patient during removal from a confined space while in a seated position and during transport.

m. A long wooden spine board with 2 - 9′ straps or other suitable substitute to permit the immobilization and transport of a spinal column fracture without vertical or horizontal expansion, contraction or twisting. (A scoop type stretcher is not a suitable substitute for this item.)

n. Blood pressure manometer, cuff and stethoscope or other suitable substitute for determining patient blood pressure both outside and inside of vehicle.

o. A poison treatment kit consisting of a minimum of 2 oz. each of activated charcoal and syrup of Ipecac or some suitable substitute for each in addition to one-half gallon potable water.

p. An obstetrical kit containing a minimum of 1 pair sterile gloves, scissors, umbilical cord clamps or tapes, sterile vaginal dressings, 2 towels, large plastic bag, and swaddling material. (Aluminum foil is acceptable as swaddling material as are burn sheets.)

q. At least two battery-operated, hand-carried portable lights.

r. Tracheal and/or esophageal intubation kits.

s. Plureal decompression kit.

t. Drugs, IV solutions, and administration kits as appropriate under regional protocol.

u. Portable cardioscope and defibrillator.

v. Biomedical telemetry communications gear to include a portable two-way radio compatible with local system.

w. Restraint devices of sufficient strength to restrain a violent adult and sufficiently padded to prevent chafing and/or injury to patient.

x. Two sets of sandbags.

D. *Combined Services*

Any designated response service which provides more than one classification (R1-R5) of service, shall meet all applicable requirements for each classification of service it provides.

E. All R2 and R5 personnel shall be required to submit a statement as to their physical and mental health on a form to be provided by the Office of Emergency Medical Services.

19-73w-402—Minimum Standards for Qualification of Personnel

The minimum standards for qualified emergency personnel are hereinafter set forth in categories for the purpose of stating the level of competence the Commissioner finds necessary for the protection of the public. The objective method adopted by the Commissioner for ascertaining the level of expertise he deems appropriate shall be a system of examinations requiring training and preparation that is set forth as follows:

A. *Medical Response Technician (MRT)*

1. A Medical Response Technician shall be a person who has:

   a. Successfully completed the state standardized Medical Response Technician written examination

      —AND—

   b. Successfully completed the state standardized Medical Response Technician practical examination.

2. To be qualified to take the above examination, a person shall have:

Successfully completed an approved CIM program
> or

Successfully completed an ARC advanced first aid and emergency care course and an approved CPR course
> or

By way of exception to these qualifications, other persons, as recommended by regional EMS councils, shall be considered qualified to take the above examinations.

3. For the purpose of maintaining a level of proficiency, an MRT must complete a Commissioner-approved 15-hour refresher course at intervals not exceeding 24 months.

4. Any person who has qualified to take the standardized examination without undergoing a Crash Injury Management (CIM) course must upon failure of the written and/or practical examination enroll in and attend an approved CIM program. Any person failing the written and/or practical examination upon completion of the CIM course shall have the opportunity for a re-examination within a 30- to 90-day period. The only exception to this time frame shall be if there is no scheduled written or practical examination within the 90-day time period.

B. *Emergency Medical Technician-Ambulance (EMT)*

1. An EMT shall be a person who has:
Successfully completed the state standardized EMT written examination
> —AND—

Successfully completed the state standardized EMT practical examination.

2. To be qualified to take the above examination, a person shall have:
Successfully completed a Commissioner-certified 81-hour EMT training program
> or

Successfully completed an ARC advanced first aid and emergency care course plus successful completion of a Commissioner-approved CPR course plus 10 hours of clinical orientation in a hospital involved in EMT training plus 6 months' active service with a state-certified R1, R2 service to include a letter of recommendation from the chief operating officer of such service
> or

Successfully completed an EMT training program which the Commissioner determines to be equivalent to state-certified EMT training or

Possession of a valid LPN, RN or MD license in the state of Connecticut plus successfully completed a Commissioner-approved extrication course

or

Successfully completed a minimum of two years' duty as a medical corpsman with a unit of the United States armed forces plus successful completion of a Commissioner-approved extrication course

or

Between 6/1/75 and 6/1/76 only, current certification of successful completion of the ARC advanced first aid (old 27 hour) course plus an AHA CPR course plus 10 hours of in-hospital clinical experience at a hospital involved with EMT training and 6 months' active service with an ambulance or rescue organization

or

Current certification as a senior national ski patroller

or

By way of exception to these qualifications, other persons as recommended by the regional EMS council shall be considered qualified to take the above examination.

3. For the purpose of maintaining a level of proficiency, an EMT must complete 25 hours of Commissioner-approved refresher training at intervals not to exceed 24 months.

4. Any person who has qualified to take the standardized examination without undergoing the Emergency Medical Technician (EMT) course must upon failure of the written and/or practical examination enroll in and attend the basic level EMT course. Any person failing the written and/or practical examination upon completion of an EMT course shall have the opportunity for a re-examination within a 30- to 90-day period. The only exception to this time frame shall be if there is no scheduled written or practical examination within the 90-day time period.

C. *Emergency Medical Technician-Advanced (EMT-II)*

1. An EMT-II shall be a person who has:
Successfully completed the state standardized EMT-II written examination

—AND—

Successfully completed the state standardized EMT-II practical examination.

2. To be qualified to take the above examinations, a person shall have:

Successfully completed a Commissioner-approved EMT-II training course

or

Successfully completed an EMT-II training course which meets or exceeds the standards defined by the Commissioner as to course content and evaluation procedures

or

Successfully completed a minimum of two years' duty as a medical corpsman with a unit of the United States armed forces and current certification as an EMT

or

Hold a current license as an RN or LPN in the state of Connecticut plus current certification as an EMT

or

Hold a current license as an MD in the state of Connecticut plus current certification as an EMT

or

By way of exception to these qualifications, other persons as recommended by regional EMS council shall be considered qualified to take the above examination.

3. For the purpose of maintaining a level of proficiency, an EMT-II must complete 20 hours of Commissioner-approved refresher training at intervals not to exceed 12 months.

4. Any person who has qualified to take the standardized examination without undergoing the Emergency Medical Technician-Advanced (EMT-II) course must upon failure of the written and/or practical examination enroll in and attend an approved EMT-II course. Any person failing the written and/or practical examination upon completion of an EMT-II course shall have the opportunity for a re-examination within a 30- to 90-day period. The only exception to this time frame shall be if there is no scheduled written or practical examination within the 90-day time period.

D. *EMS Instructor*

1. An EMS Instructor shall be a person who has:
   a. Current state certification as an EMT.
   b. A minimum of one year active involvement with an ambulance or rescue organization or in the EMS care field.
   c. A letter of recommendation from the EMS council for the region or regions in which he or she shall act as an instructor. Such letter must be as the result of a motion brought before such council/councils for a quorum vote as the result of a letter of recommendation from an

Emergency Room physician within the region and the chief operating officer of the EMS organization with which the individual serves.

    d. Successfully completed a Commissioner-approved EMS Instructor's course or its equivalent as approved by OEMS.

    e. By way of exception to "d" above, other persons as recommended by the regional EMS council shall be considered for a waiver based upon criteria to be established by the Connecticut Advisory Committee on Emergency Medical Services.

  2. For the purpose of maintaining a level of proficiency, an EMS Instructor must complete 25 hours of Commissioner-approved refresher training at intervals not exceeding 24 months.

E. *Equivalency*

The following shall be considered automatic equivalency with no additional documentation required.

  1. EMT-II equivalent to EMT and MRT.

  2. EMS Instructor equivalent to EMT and MRT.

  3. EMT equivalent to MRT.

19-73w-403—Minimum Standards—Vehicles

Intent: In order to insure conformance to vehicle design and equipment regulations without undue inconvenience to providers, this section provides for an easy method of determination that a vehicle is current in certification by means of an exterior identification. It additionally provides a readily identifiable assurance to a patient that he/she is in competent hands by virtue of interior identification.

A. *R2 vehicles* shall be inspected as often as necessary to insure conformance to regulations but at least annually by OEMS or their designated agent for design and equipment conformance for vehicle safety commencing 1/1/77.

B. As of 1/1/77 each such R2 vehicle shall display decals on the rear exterior and in the patient compartment of such vehicle indicating it is certified by OEMS as an R2 vehicle. Such decal must be easily visible from the patient compartment and the exterior, rear of said vehicle.

C. Each R2 certified vehicle shall be licensed by the Connecticut Department of Motor Vehicles as an "ambulance."

D. Any vehicle routinely used to respond to medical emergencies for the purpose of supplying medical assistance and patient transportation shall be certified in conformance with these regulations.

E. Upon successful completion of the inspections stipulated above, such vehicle shall be certified by OEMS and a decal affixed to the rear exterior of such vehicle so indicating. Such decal shall be easily visible from the rear, exterior of said vehicle.

F. Any certified response service which is aggrieved by the results of such inspection, may within 30 days from date of inspection, file a complaint with the Director OEMS, and a hearing shall be held within 30 days of receipt of such complaint.

19-73w-404—Service Standards

Intent: In order to eliminate existing problems concerning stacking of emergency calls, rotation lists, lack of accountability, etc., this section creates a system of specifically assigned responsibility for all geographic areas in the state. Additionally, variance from this assigned responsibility is allowable only with the full understanding and agreement of parties involved.

A. *Response Services*

  1. All response services shall make application for designation to the OEMS in a form and manner prescribed by that Office indicating:

    a. Such service is a duly incorporated agency under Connecticut law, and there is a chief operating officer, who shall be indicated, and who shall sign the application for certification and who is specifically accountable for the EMS operations of such agency

        or

    b. Such agency is a duly designated element of a governmental body which has a chief executive officer, who shall be indicated, and who shall sign the application, and a responsible officer of the agency who shall be directly responsible for EMS activities who shall also sign the application.

  2. Such responder shall:

    a. Respond to calls for EMS originating from the EMS dispatch center for their Primary Service Area (PSA) on a 24-hour, 7-day a week basis or enclose a copy of a written agreement with other certified response services which offer coverage for their PSA during non-operational hours with no substantial reduction in quality of service or increase in response time.

  b. Notify dispatcher and/or caller at time of dispatch or call if a unit is not immediately available to respond.

  c. Maintain records, in a form and manner prescribed by the Director OEMS, of each emergency response.

  d. Maintain contact with central dispatch center concerning location of system vehicles any time such vehicles are at other location than normal duty station (i.e., maintenance, meals, routine transfers, etc.).

  e. Have been assigned a PSA.

 3. Any service which is being established for the first time in Connecticut shall meet all requirements which would be applicable on 1/1/77.

B. *Assignment of Primary Service Area (PSA)*

 1. A PSA shall be assigned, in writing, by the EMS planning agency for the region(s) in which such PSA lies. Such assignment shall be approved/disapproved by the Commissioner. Such written assignment shall be in a form and manner prescribed by OEMS and shall include number of vehicles to be certified for use within such PSA.

 2. A PSA shall be assigned to only one designated response service for a given category (R1, R2 & R5) of service. Any circumstances under which another designated response service would receive first-call priority (such as central dispatch sending closest available vehicle) shall be stipulated in a written response plan for Emergency Medical Services.

19-73w-405—EMS Paraprofessional Training Program
Approval Criteria

A. In order to conduct a state-approved Emergency Medical Service Paraprofessional Training Program, an organization must:

 1. Make written application to conduct training to the Commissioner in a form and manner prescribed by that Commissioner. Such form shall include, but not be limited to:

  a. Approval of the regional EMS council where training shall be conducted.

  b. A listing of the teaching facilities to be used, the availability of teaching aids and supplies.

  c. A list of instructors, assistant instructors, and physician lecturers to be used during the course of the program.

 2. Provide for continuous supervision of the program by a state-certified EMS Instructor.

 3. Follow guidelines for training established by the Commissioner.

  4. Maintain financial and administrative records for inspection as required by the Commissioner.
B. Emergency Medical Technician Program Enrollment Criteria
  1. In order to be enrolled in a state-approved Emergency Medical Technician program, an individual must make application to the agency conducting the program in a form and manner approved by the Director OEMS. Such applicant must be 18 years of age* or over, and fall within one of the following categories:
      a. Be affiliated with a designated R2 response service.
      b. Be affiliated with a rescue service.
      c. Be affiliated with a designated R1 response service.
      d. Be affiliated with a police or fire service.
      e. All others.
    Such applicant will be chosen according to the priorities listed above, letter *a* being the highest.
NOTE: *Special exceptions to the 18-year age minimum will be considered by the Commissioner if such applicant is affiliated with a designated R1, R2 or R5 response service.

19-73w-406—Prohibited Acts
The following shall be prohibited:
A. The possession or carrying of dangerous or concealed weapons on or in an emergency medical service vehicle or by any person functioning as an emergency medical service provider except that sworn police officers may carry dangerous or concealed weapons in the performance of their duties as they relate to said emergency medical service vehicles.
B. The possession of handcuffs or other restraint devices not approved for use by OEMS except by sworn police officers in the performance of their duties.
C. Smoking in the patient compartment of any emergency medical service vehicle.
D. Any act which is detrimental to the safety and welfare of a patient or the general public as determined by OEMS under the provisions of Chapter 54 of the Connecticut General Statutes as amended.

19-73w-407—Exceptions
Where an individual or service feels that any of these regulations have been incorrectly or unfairly applied, that individual or service shall have the right to ask that the appropriate regional EMS council hear the complaint and respond to it within 30 days. Where a regional

council feels that any of these regulations have been incorrectly or unfairly applied in an individual or service case, that regional council shall have the right to ask that the Commissioner hear the complaint and respond to it within 60 days. The Commissioner and the Advisory Committee shall be advised in writing. This shall not waive the right of an individual or individual service to directly appeal to the Commissioner a regional council decision unfavorable to them.

Be it known that the within and foregoing rules and regulations are made, adopted and promulgated by the undersigned pursuant to Section 19-73W(e) of the General Statutes after publication in the Connecticut Law Journal on July 15, 1975 of the notice of the proposal to adopt them and the holding of advertised public hearings during July and August 1975, on the issuance thereof and after consideration of all relevant matter presented are added to the rules and regulations of this Department, pertaining to EMS Transportation Services, and the training of Emergency Medical Services personnel.

In Witness Whereof, I have hereunto set my hand and seal this 22nd day of September 1975.

DOUGLAS S. LLOYD, M.D.
Commissioner of Health

Appendix 11D

Report of Findings and Recommendations for a Categorization System for Hospital Emergency Service Capability in Connecticut (October 1975)*

Task Force on Categorization:
G. Strauch, M.D., Chairman
A. Brandt, M.D.
E. Browne, M.D.
T. Krizek, M.D.
A. Penttieri, M.D.
H. Goldberg, R.N.
R. Bergeron
S. Webb

Resource Persons to Task Force:
E. O'Gara
J. Cannon

*As modified and approved by the Connecticut Advisory Committee on Emergency Medical Services (February 9, 1976)

Accreditation and Categorization of Emergency Departments:
The current dictum that an ambulance should deliver a patient to the nearest emergency unit is no longer acceptable. It is essential that road maps and road signs, at appropriate locations, designate routes to hospitals and emergency departments. The patient must be transported to the emergency department best prepared for this particular problem. In the absence of a descriptive categorization of the level of care that might reasonably be expected at a facility, neither the patient nor the ambulance driver can judge which facility is adequate to the immediate need. It is usually taken for granted by the general public that every emergency room can render full care for injuries of all magnitudes. There is the obligation to the severely injured patient as well as to the lone physician, to the small staffs of remote hospitals, and to institutions with minimal emergency department facilities, that the public be thoroughly informed of the extent of care that can be administered at emergency departments of varying levels of competence. A categorization of emergency departments would serve to indicate the level of care that a patient might reasonably expect.

—*Accidental Death and Disability: The Neglected Disease of Modern Society,* prepared by the Division of Medical Sciences, National Academy of Sciences and National Research Council, Committees on Trauma and Shock, Division of Medical Sciences, National Academy of Sciences, National Research Council. No. 1071-A-13, September 1966.

STATEMENT OF HISTORY AND INTENT

From the late 1960s to the present, concern for quality emergency care has been reflected by increased research efforts, planning and legislative activity aimed at improving emergency medical services. In many communities, the loose collection of transportation, communication, physician and hospital services have been closely examined. The effectiveness of the organization and coordination of these services has become the subject for debate among professional organizations, as well as a concern of interested citizens.

Three major alternatives for improving the response of emergency departments to the emergency victim have been recommended most often. These alternatives include upgrading of emergency departments, categorization of emergency departments and regionalization of emergency departments.

It has been the purpose of this effort to explore the categorization process. The basic philosophy of categorization suggests that emergency departments should be systematized according to their current level of capability, rather than have every facility attempt to attain the same level of capability. Because it would be financially impossible and economically unsound to staff and equip all emergency departments as major trauma and medical centers, categorization, as seen by its proponents, should:

(1) Encourage the proper performance of emergency care by properly trained individuals in a proper environment;
(2) Prevent duplication of specialized services within the emergency care system;
(3) Improve the capabilities of hospitals to provide effective emergency care for all patients served by the hospital.

In November, 1973 Public Law 93-154 was signed by the President. As part of the requirements determined by the Department of Health, Education and Welfare for the implementation of this law, each state has been requested to develop a categorization of its emergency facilities. In August, 1974 the state of Connecticut adopted Public Act 74-305. Through this Act the Commission on Hospitals and Health Care was charged with the development and coordination of a statewide emergency medical services system. This Act defined the powers and duties of the Commission and Regional Councils, as they relate to EMS. Since May, 1975 the responsibilities and duties for implementation of this law have been transferred by the Connecticut Legislature to the Office of Emergency Medical Services of the Department of Health of the State.

There has been general agreement among those concerned with the EMS development in Connecticut that if there is to be an effective change in emergency activities, analysis of data pertaining to the entire emergency medical care system must be undertaken. While there exists in Connecticut and elsewhere available data on communication and transportation services, there is an urgent need to consider hospital and physician services, the diagnostic mix of patient load in the emergency department, the cost of delivery of emergency medical care, the effect of emergency department activities on hospital in-patient services and the legal implications to the hospital for the operation of emergency departments. The Yale Trauma Program Study of Emergency Medical Facilities in Connecticut, released in 1973, recommended categorization of hospital emergency services. In January, 1974 the Connecticut Chapter of the American College of Surgeons, in conjunction with the Connecticut State Medical Society, undertook to study and analyze the capabilities of emergency departments in Connecticut's short-term acute general hospitals. One of the purposes of that study was to recommend a practical system for identifying and defining emergency department capabilities in Connecticut. Those responsible for the study recognized that categorization of emergency facilities would require further analysis and assistance from medical professionals in order to be realistic and acceptable.

Professional involvement in accumulating facts, developing alternative systems and evaluating the effects of these systems is paramount to the success of future EMS systems, and, in particular, of emergency department categorization.

In January, 1975, the Director of the Division of Emergency Medical Services of the Commission on Hospitals and Health Care in Connecticut, in response to the H.E.W. request for categorization of emergency departments, asked that the Chairman of the Connecticut Committee on Trauma of the American College of Surgeons undertake such a categorization. The Chairman invited representatives of several organizations recognized as critical to the categorization development in Connecticut to participate in this endeavor. It was felt that this work could provide the critical element of medical/professional involvement in categorization, as its most important contribution.

The membership of the Task Force includes:

Gerald O. Strauch, M.D., F.A.C.S., Chairman
1. Chairman, Connecticut Committee on Trauma, American College of Surgeons
2. President Elect, Connecticut Society of American Board of Surgeons
3. Vice-Chairman, Connecticut State Medical Society Committee on Emergency Medical Services and Accident Prevention
4. Member, Board of Directors, American Trauma Society, Connecticut Division
5. Member, Ad Hoc Connecticut Advisory Committee on Emergency Medical Services

Allan A. Brandt, M.D.
1. President, Connecticut Chapter of American College of Emergency Physicians
2. Member, Connecticut State Medical Society Committee on Emergency Medical Services and Accident Prevention
3. Member, Connecticut State Committee on Cardio-Pulmonary Resuscitation and Emergency Cardiac Care
4. Member, Ad Hoc Connecticut Advisory Committee on Emergency Medical Services

Edward R. Brown, M.D.
1. Chairman, Connecticut State Medical Society Committee on Emergency Medical Services and Accident Prevention
2. Former President, Connecticut Chapter of American College of Emergency Physicians
3. Member, Connecticut Advisory Committee on Emergency Medical Services
4. Member, Ad Hoc Connecticut Advisory Committee on Emergency Medical Services

Thomas J. Krizek, M.D., F.A.C.S.
1. President, Connecticut Chapter of American College of Surgeons
2. Member and Former Chairman, Connecticut Committee on Trauma, American College of Surgeons
3. Committee on Trauma, American College of Surgeons
4. Member, Connecticut Advisory Committee on Emergency Medical Services
5. Director, Yale Trauma Program
6. Member, Board of Directors, American Trauma Society, Connecticut Division
7. Member, Ad Hoc Connecticut Advisory Committee on Emergency Medical Services

Andrew J. Panettieri, M.D., F.A.C.S.
1. Former President, Connecticut Chapter of American College of Surgeons
2. President and Member, Board of Directors, American Trauma Society, Connecticut Division
3. Member, Connecticut Committee on Trauma, American College of Surgeons
4. Member, American Burn Association

Helen Goldberg, R.N.
1. President, Connecticut Chapter, Emergency Department Nurses Association
2. Member, Connecticut Advisory Committee on Emergency Medical Services
3. Member, Subcommittee on Categorization, Connecticut Advisory Committee on Emergency Medical Services

Robert D. Bergeron
1. Member, Connecticut Advisory Committee on Emergency Medical Services

2. Chairman, Subcommittee on Categorization, Connecticut Advisory Committee on Emergency Medical Services
3. Vice-President, Education, Connecticut Hospital Association
4. Co-Chairman, Ad Hoc Connecticut Advisory Committee on Emergency Medical Services

Samuel B. Webb, Jr., Dr. P.H.
1. Co-Project Director, 1973 Report to the Governor of Connecticut by the Yale Trauma Program
2. Director, Yale Hospital Administration Program
3. Associate Member and Secretary, Connecticut Committee on Trauma, American College of Surgeons
4. Member, Ad Hoc Connecticut Advisory Committee on Emergency Medical Services

RESOURCE PERSONS TO TASK FORCE:

Eileen M. O'Gara, M.P.H.
Research Assistant to Connecticut Committee on Trauma, American College of Surgeons

Joseph F. Cannon, M.P.H.
Co-Director, Yale Trauma Program

The Task Force had its first meeting in February, 1975. It is important to note that it has received the full cooperation of the Office of Emergency Medical Services of the State Department of Health since it began its work. The initial task undertaken was to develop a categorization scheme appropriate for the state of Connecticut. For the purpose of these recommendations, an emergency service facility or emergency department refers only to those services maintained by the short-term acute general hospitals in Connecticut. Although other institutions provide types of emergency services, it was decided early in the planning stages of these considerations that because the short term acute general hospital emergency departments represent such a large percentage of the total volume that the initial phase of categorization should be limited to them. While the other institutions are a valuable community resource, and should be included in developing disaster or other contingency plans, they offer limited accessibility and should not be considered primary providers of emergency medical care for the at-large population of the state.

As the work of the Task Force proceeded, it became clear to its members that a categorization process which limited itself to criteria related only to the Emergency Room or Department would ignore the essential nature of the impact of other hospital resources on the delivery of emergency care. Therefore, the Task Force members agreed to present these recommendations as criteria for examining the emergency service capability of the institutions. The impact of all of the essential resources of the institutions has to be a paramount consideration in establishing emergency services capability.

Based on the process developed as a result of this decision, the Task Force began to examine data related to Connecticut hospitals. Data utilized in this examination included:

1. American Hospital Association, *The Hospital Emergency Department in an Emergency Care System*, The Association, Chicago, 1972;
2. American College of Surgeons Committee on Trauma, *Guidelines for Design and Function of a Hospital Emergency Department*, Chicago, 1971;
3. Hospital Council of Southern California, *Guidelines for Hospital Emergency Services*, 1971;
4. Yale Trauma Program, *Recommendations from a Report to the Governor*, 1973;
5. *Categorization of Emergency Departments in Connecticut's 35 Short-Term General Hospitals: A Feasibility Study*, Eileen O'Gara, M.P.H., 1975;
6. American Hospital Association, *The American Hospital Association Guide to the Health Care Field*, 1974; and
7. American Medical Association, *The Directory of Approved Internship and Residency Programs, 1974–1975*.

The personal knowledge of the members of the Task Force also proved to be an essential resource. However, the contributions and impact of many persons must be noted. Often, the recognition of individual efforts is unknown or unnoticed. Clearly, the Task Force owes a great deal to individuals and organizations who have committed themselves to the improvement of emergency medical services. We have attempted to bring to bear the professional judgment necessary to create the first categorization for Emergency Service Capability in Connecticut. We have pride in our accomplishment for its value as a realistic and comprehensive starting point for full consideration and implementation of a categorization system in Connecticut.

STATEMENT OF PURPOSE AND USE

This categorization system is designed to identify the essential man-power, facilities, equipment and organizational elements necessary for the existence of an adequate emergency medical services delivery capability in Connecticut hospitals. It is organized to define four levels of capability:

> Standard Emergency Service
> Major Emergency Service
> Comprehensive Emergency Service
> Limited Emergency Service[a]

It should identify those hospitals capable of rendering resuscitative and supportive patient management, until transfer may be effected in special types of cases; others capable of definitive care for all but the most unusual problems, and those capable of rendering emergency medical care of the highest sophistication.

It is expected that this categorization system will be used to review and to adequately determine the most appropriate facility to which the patient may be taken by emergency vehicles.

Hospitals may also wish to use this categorization information as a self-reviewed tool to determine the capability of their own emergency services.

The Task Force *does not* believe that this categorization system can or should be used as a singular tool to assess the quality of emergency care in any setting, but rather that it will allow providers to more clearly examine their own needs and capabilities.

---

[a]Following the development of criteria for the first three categories listed below, discussions among Task Force members and between the Task Force, several hospitals, and other relevant organizations seemed to mandate definition of another possible category. The reason for establishing such a category is the possibility that one or more hospitals may not conform to other categories. Since the Task Force believes that the cornerstone of the Connecticut categorization system should be the Standard Category defined herein, it was decided to designate as a Limited Emergency Service any emergency service which meets the minimum criteria contained in the Appendix (see *Minimum Emergency Service Criteria*), but does not conform to any of the three other categories.

The Limited Emergency Service is a service that for one reason or another may be capable of treating many individuals with real or apparent emergency medical conditions; however, it does not conform to the criteria established for the Standard Emergency Service.

STANDARD EMERGENCY SERVICE

The Standard Emergency Service is capable of treating most individuals with real or apparent emergency medical conditions. In certain instances of critical illness or injury, definitive treatment may require transfer of the patient to another facility after initial evaluation and preliminary resuscitation.

I. Emergency Department Characteristics
   A. Access to Hospital-Emergency Department Complex
      1. Identification of and access to hospital (2–5 miles)
         a. Directional signs from highway to hospital
         b. Signs posted on streets adjacent to hospital and main streets leading to hospital
         c. Directional signs on hospital property designating Emergency Department entrance
         d. Emergency Department accessible to ground transportation in all types of weather
      2. Access to Emergency Department
         a. Restricted parking near Emergency Department entrance
         b. Clearly marked entrance
         c. Separate outside entrance
         d. Ground level entrance
         e. Clearance for more than one vehicle
         f. Unloading platform
         g. Overhead coverage for ambulance unloading area
         h. Doors to permit easy passage of stretchers, wheelchairs, IV equipment
   B. Staffing
      1. 24 hour staffing by a physician(s) capable of managing surgical and nonsurgical emergencies with no additional hospital duties during period of Emergency Department duty
      2. 24 hour Emergency Department staffing by regularly assigned registered nurses
      3. 24 hour availability of attendants capable of assisting in listing or otherwise transporting patients from one place to another
   C. Plant Layout
      1. Specifically designated areas
         a. Registration
         b. Patient waiting area

     c. Examination and treatment rooms
     d. Minor surgery rooms
     e. Physicians' and nurses' work areas
     f. Equipment storage
  2. Separate and/or partitioned rooms for treatment of individual patients
  3. Appropriate Emergency Department illumination
  4. Auxiliary power provisions

D. Equipment
  1. Medications and supplies required for most common emergency problems
  2. Sterile surgical sets
  3. Splints
  4. Thoracic and abdominal paracentesis sets
  5. Intravenous fluids and administration devices
  6. Suction devices
  7. Gastric lavage equipment
  8. Mechanical ventilator
  9. Intubation tray
  10. Trachestomy tray
  11. Catheterization tray
  12. Wall or portable oxygen
  13. Electrocardiograph
  14. Cardiac monitor-defibrillator
  15. Central venous monitoring setups
  16. Pacemakers
  17. Closed thoracostomy tray
  18. Wheelchairs
  19. Stretchers

E. Policies
  1. Medical direction and accountability for the Emergency Department by a physician/director
  2. Written procedures for the procurement of equipment and medications
  3. Open 24 hours a day
  4. Medical records maintained on all patients
  5. Protocol for notification of a patient's family and personal physician as established by hospital staff
  6. Patients accepted for treatment without regard to race, creed, sex, color or determination of ability to pay
  7. All physicians employed in Emergency Department certified according to latest American Heart Association Advanced Life Support procedures

8. All employed personnel engaged in care of patients in Emergency Department certified according to latest American Heart Association Basic Life Support procedures as a prerequisite for employment

9. Emergency Department references regarding tetanus, burn, wounds and other emergency problems

10. Predetermined plan for diagnosis and treatment of the alcoholic or drug abuse patient

11. Regular audit of records

12. Continuing Education Program for all Emergency Department Personnel

13. Maintenance of poison control index and communication with Poison Control Center

14. System for patient follow-up care as established by hospital medical staff

15. Communications with other municipal, state, and federal health agencies

F. Communications

1. Telephone in Emergency Department with separate outside line

2. Intra-hospital communication by telephone

3. Direct two-way radio communication with ambulance

4. Direct two-way radio communication with central EMS dispatcher

II. Characteristics of Hospital Operating an Emergency Department

A. Backup Medical Staffing

1. *Available Within 20 Minutes* of notification, under normal conditions and circumstances.
   a. Anesthesiologist
   b. Cardiologist
   c. General Surgeon
   d. Internist
   e. Obstetrician
   f. Orthopedic Surgeon
   g. Pediatrician

2. *Available Within 60 Minutes* of notification, under normal conditions and circumstances.
   a. Otolaryngologist
   b. Radiologist
   c. Urologist

B. Physical Plant

1. Medical-surgical ICU-CCU having the capacity to give at least initial intensive care to all types of patients

with emergencies commonly requiring such units, staffed 24 hours

2. Operating rooms available with 24 hour staffing
3. Blood bank within the facility (a medical facility within the hospital, staffed by qualified technicians and under the medical direction of a physician capable of and responsible for the procurement, drawing, processing, storage and distribution of whole blood and plasma)
4. Postoperative recovery area available 24 hours and staffed whenever patients are present
5. Central sterile supply room
6. Delivery suite available, with staffing, within 30 minutes of notice
7. Hospital switchboard—open 24 hours
8. Admitting Office
9. Medical records department
10. Morgue

C. Support Services (available, 24 hours)
1. Proctoscopy
2. Bronchoscopy
3. Radiology (plain, contrast and scintiscan studies)
4. Laboratory (for indispensable laboratory tests related to emergency medical problems)
5. Blood bank
6. Respiratory therapy

D. Policies
1. Specific definition of administration of Emergency Department
2. General written policies as guides for Emergency Department personnel
3. Emergency Department record incorporated into the patient's hospital record
4. Admitting office representative available 24 hours
5. Ready access by emergency department to other space, equipment, supplies and drugs
6. Written Disaster Plan with periodic drills
7. Job descriptions
8. Protocol for securing cardio-pulmonary bypass for patients for whom it is required
9. 24-hour availability of representative of hospital administration

MAJOR EMERGENCY SERVICE

A Major Emergency Service can perform all the functions of a Standard Emergency Service. In addition, its manpower and/or service capabilities allow treatment of all but the most unusual emergency conditions or the accommodation of larger numbers of individuals in a given period of time.

I. Emergency Department Characteristics
  A. Access to Hospital-Emergency Department Complex
    1. Identification of and access to hospital (2-5 miles)
      a. Directional signs from highway to hospital
      b. Signs posted on streets adjacent to hospital and main streets leading to hospital
      c. Directional signs on hospital property designating Emergency Department entrance
      d. Emergency Department accessible to ground transportation in all types of weather
    2. Access to Emergency Department
      a. Restricted parking near Emergency Department entrance
      b. Clearly marked entrance
      c. Separate outside entrance
      d. Ground level entrance
      e. Clearance for more than one vehicle
      f. Unloading platform
      g. Overhead coverage for ambulance unloading area
      h. Doors to permit easy passage of stretchers, wheelchairs, IV equipment
  B. Staffing
    1. 24 hour staffing by a physician capable of managing surgical and nonsurgical emergencies with no additional hospital duties during period of Emergency duty
    2. 24 hour Emergency Department staffing by regularly assigned registered nurses
    3. 24 hour availability of attendants capable of assisting in lifting or otherwise transporting patients from one place to another
    4. Staffing by two physicians simultaneously to accommodate additional patient care needs, according to an established hospital plan.

C. Plant Layout
   1. Specifically designated areas
      a. Registration
      b. Patient waiting area
      c. Examination and treatment rooms
      d. Minor surgery rooms
      e. Physicians' and nurses' work areas
      f. Equipment storage
   2. Separate and/or partitioned rooms for treatment of individual patients
   3. Appropriate Emergency Department illumination
   4. Auxiliary power provisions
   5. Radiologic facility, in or adjacent to Emergency Department, for plain films, contrast studies
   6. Plaster room
   7. Observation area
   8. Doctor's on-call room
   9. Storage for Emergency Department housekeeping supplies
  10. Waiting room visible from entrance to Emergency Department
  11. Patient registration area
      a. Visible from nurses' work area
      b. Visible from waiting room
      c. Visible from entrance
      d. Has accessible communications with nurses' work area
  12. Ambulance entrance visible from nurses' work area
D. Equipment
   1. Medications and supplies required for most common emergency problems
   2. Sterile surgical sets
   3. Splints
   4. Thoracic and abdominal paracentesis sets
   5. Intravenous fluids and administration devices
   6. Suction devices
   7. Gastric lavage equipment
   8. Mechanical ventilator
   9. Intubation tray
  10. Tracheostomy tray
  11. Catheterization tray
  12. Wall or portable oxygen
  13. Electrocardiograph

14. Cardiac monitor-defibrillator
15. Central venous monitoring setups
16. Pacemakers
17. Closed thoracostomy tray
18. Wheelchairs
19. Stretchers

E. Policies
1. Medical direction and accountability for the Emergency Department by a physician-director
2. Written procedures for the procurement of equipment and medications
3. Open 24 hours a day
4. Medical records maintained on all patients
5. Protocol for notification of a patient's family and personal physician as established by hospital staff
6. Patients accepted for treatment without regard to race, creed, sex, color or determination of ability to pay
7. All physicians employed in Emergency Department certified according to latest American Heart Association Advanced Life Support procedures
8. All employed personnel engaged in care of patients in Emergency Department certified according to latest American Heart Association Basic Life Support procedures as a prerequisite for employment
9. Emergency Department references regarding tetanus, burn, wounds and other emergency problems
10. Predetermined plan for diagnosis and treatment of the alcoholic or drug abuse patient
11. Regular audit of records
12. Continuing Education Program for all Emergency Department Personnel
13. Maintenance of poison control index and communication with Poison Control Center
14. System for patient follow-up care as established by hospital medical staff
15. Communications with other municipal, state, and federal health agencies

F. Communications
1. Telephone in Emergency Department with separate outside line
2. Intra-hospital communication by telephone
3. Direct two-way radio communication with ambulance

    4. Direct two-way radio communication with central EMS dispatcher

    5. Telephone in doctor's on-call room

    6. Direct communication with key staff

    7. Direct communication with police

    8. Direct two-way communication with other key hospitals

II. Characteristics of Hospital Operating an Emergency Department

    A. Backup Medical Staffing

        1. *Available Within 20 Minutes* of notification, under normal conditions and circumstances.

            a. Anesthesiologist

            b. Cardiologist

            c. General Surgeon

            d. Internist

            e. Obstetrician

            f. Orthopedic Surgeon

            g. Pediatrician

            h. Neurosurgeon

            i. Thoracic Surgeon

            j. Ophthalmologist

            k. Otolaryngologist

        2. *Available Within 60 Minutes* of notification, under normal conditions and circumstances.

            a. Radiologist

            b. Urologist

            c. Chest Disease Specialist

            d. Psychiatrist

    B. Physical Plant

        1. Medical-surgical ICU-CCU having the capacity to give at least initial intensive care to all types of patients with emergencies commonly requiring such units, staffed 24 hours

        2. Operating rooms available with 24 hour staffing

        3. Blood bank within the facility (a medical facility within the hospital, staffed by qualified technicians and under the medical direction of a physician capable of and responsible for the procurement, drawing, processing, storage and distribution of whole blood and plasma)

        4. Postoperative recovery area available 24 hours and staffed whenever patients are present

        5. Central sterile supply room

6. Delivery suite with 24-hour in-house staffing within 30 minutes of notice
7. Hospital switchboard—open 24 hours
8. Admitting Office
9. Medical records department
10. Morgue
11. In-patient psychiatric beds

C. Support Services (available 24 hours)
1. Proctoscopy
2. Bronchoscopy
3. Radiology (plain, contrast and scintiscan studies)
4. Laboratory (for indispensable laboratory tests related to emergency medical problems)
5. Blood bank
6. Respiratory Therapy
7. Esophagogastroscopy
8. Angiography
9. Burn service
10. Peritoneal dialysis
11. Inpatient psychiatry
12. Nuclear medicine
13. Echoencephalography
14. Anesthesia
15. Postoperative recovery facilities

D. Policies
1. Specific definition of adminstration of Emergency Department
2. General written policies as guides for Emergency Department personnel
3. Emergency Department record incorporated into the patient's hospital record
4. Admitting office representative available 24 hours
5. Ready access by Emergency Department to other space, equipment, supplies and drugs
6. Written Disaster Plan with periodic drills
7. Job descriptions
8. Protocol for securing cardio-pulmonary bypass for patients for whom it is required
9. Previous medical records promptly available to Emergency Department staff
10. 24-hour availability of representative of hospital administration

COMPREHENSIVE EMERGENCY SERVICE

A Comprehensive Emergency Service can perform all the functions of a Major Emergency Service.

A Comprehensive Emergency Service's capability extends to provision of definitive treatment of all individuals with any real or apparent emergency medical condition, except under extraordinary circumstances (*e.g.*, disaster).

I. Emergency Department Characteristics
    A. Access to Hospital-Emergency Department Complex
        1. Identification of and access to hospital (2–5 miles)
            a. Directional signs from highway to hospital
            b. Signs posted on streets adjacent to hospital and main streets leading to hospital
            c. Directional signs on hospital property designating Emergency Department entrance
            d. Emergency Department accessible to ground transportation in all types of weather
        2. Access to Emergency Department
            a. Restricted parking near Emergency Department entrance
            b. Clearly marked entrance
            c. Separate outside entrance
            d. Ground level entrance
            e. Clearance for more than one vehicle
            f. Unloading platform
            g. Overhead coverage for ambulance unloading area
            h. Doors to permit easy passage of stretchers, wheelchairs, IV equipment
    B. Staffing
        1. Institutionally based medical director
        2. 24 hour Emergency Department staffing by regularly assigned registered nurses
        3. 24 hour availability of attendants capable of assisting in lifting or otherwise transporting patients from one place to another
        4. 24 hour Emergency Department staffing by two physicians capable of managing surgical and non-surgical emergencies
    C. Plant Layout
        1. Specifically designated areas
            a. Registration

   b. Patient waiting area
   c. Examination and treatment rooms
   d. Minor surgery rooms
   e. Physicians' and nurses' work areas
   f. Equipment storage
2. Separate and/or partitioned rooms for treatment of individual patients
3. Appropriate Emergency Department illumination
4. Auxiliary power provisions
5. Plaster room
6. Doctor's on-call room
7. Storage for Emergency Department housekeeping supplies
8. Waiting room visible from entrance to Emergency Department
9. Patient registration area
   a. Visible from nurses' work area
   b. Visible from waiting room
   c. Visible from entrance
   d. Has accessible communications with nurses' work area
10. Ambulance entrance visible from nurses' work area
11. Radiologic facility, in or adjacent to Emergency Department, for plain films, contrast studies
12. Holding and observation area
13. Quiet room
14. Separation of critically ill patients
15. Designated press, police and ambulance attendants areas
16. Isolation unit
17. Fully equipped operating room in or adjacent to the Emergency Department

D. Equipment
1. Medications and supplies required for the most common emergency problems
2. Sterile surgical sets
3. Splints
4. Thoracic and abdominal paracentesis sets
5. Intravenous fluids and administration devices
6. Suction devices
7. Gastric lavage equipment
8. Mechanical ventilator
9. Intubation tray

    10. Tracheostomy tray
    11. Catheterization tray
    12. Wall or portable oxygen
    13. Electrocardiograph
    14. Cardiac monitor-defibrillator
    15. Central venous monitoring setups
    16. Pacemakers
    17. Closed thoracostomy tray
    18. Wheelchairs
    19. Stretchers
    20. Autoclave

E. Policies
1. Written procedures for the procurement of equipment and medications
2. Open 24 hours a day
3. Medical records maintained on all patients
4. Protocol for notification of a patient's family and personal physician as established by hospital and medical staff
5. Patients accepted for treatment without regard to race, creed, color, sex or determination of ability to pay
6. All physicians employed in Emergency Department certified according to latest American Heart Association Advanced Life Support procedures
7. All employed personnel engaged in care of patients in Emergency Department certified according to latest American Heart Association Basic Life Support procedures as a prerequisite for employment
8. Emergency Department references regarding tetanus, burn, wounds and other emergency problems
9. Predetermined plan for diagnosis and treatment of the alcoholic or drug abuse patient
10. Regular audit of records
11. Continuing Education Program for all Emergency Department Personnel
12. Maintenance of poison control index and communication with Poison Control Center
13. System for patient follow-up care as established by hospital medical staff
14. Radiation decontamination protocol
15. Communications with other municipal, state, and federal health agencies

   F. Communications
1. Telephone with separate outside line
2. Intra-hospital communication by telephone
3. Direct two-way radio communication with ambulance
4. Direct two-way radio communication with central EMS dispatcher
5. Telephone in doctor's on-call room
6. Direct communication with key staff
7. Direct communication with police
8. Direct two-way radio communication with other key hospitals

II. Characteristics of Hospital Operating an Emergency Department
   A. Backup Medical Staffing
1. *Available Within 10 Minutes* of notification, under normal conditions and circumstances.
   a. Anesthesiologist
   b. Cardiologist
   c. General Surgeon
   d. Internist
   e. Neurosurgeon
   f. Orthopedic Surgeon
   g. Pediatrician
   h. Psychiatrist
   i. Radiologist
   j. Thoracic Surgeon
2. *Available Within 20 Minutes* of notification, under normal conditions and circumstances.
   a. Obstetrician
   b. Ophthalmologist
   c. Otolaryngologist
   d. Plastic Surgeon
3. *Available Within 60 Minutes* of notification, under normal conditions and circumstances.
   a. Urologist
   b. Chest Disease Specialist

   B. Physical Plant
1. Medical-surgical ICU-CCU having the capacity to give at least initial intensive care to all types of patients with emergencies commonly requiring such units, staffed 24 hours
2. Operating rooms available with 24-hour staffing
3. Blood bank within the facility (a medical facility within the hospital, staffed by qualified technicians

and under the medical direction of a physician capable of and responsible for the procurement, drawing, processing, storage and distribution of whole blood and plasma)

4. Postoperative recovery area available 24 hours and staffed whenever patients are present
5. Delivery suite with 24-hour in-house staffing
6. Hospital switchboard—open 24 hours
7. Admitting Office
8. Medical records department
9. Morgue
10. Inpatient psychiatric beds
11. Poison control center, information immediately available
12. Pharmacy
13. Pediatric intensive care capability
14. Otolaryngology room
15. Specific provisions for management of patients with major burns

C. Support Services (available, 24 hours)
1. Proctoscopy
2. Bronchoscopy
3. Radiology (plain, contrast and scintiscan studies)
4. Laboratory (for indispensable laboratory tests related to emergency medical problems)
5. Blood bank
6. Esophagogastroscopy
7. Angiography
8. Burn service
9. Peritoneal dialysis
10. Inpatient psychiatry
11. Nuclear medicine
12. Echoencephalography
13. Anesthesia
14. Postoperative recovery facilities
15. Ultrasound
16. Respiratory therapy

D. Policies
1. Specific definition of administration of Emergency Department
2. General written policies as guides for Emergency Department personnel

3. Emergency Department record incorporated into the patient's hospital record
4. Admitting office representative available 24 hours
5. Ready access by Emergency Department to other space, equipment, supplies and drugs
6. Written Disaster Plan with periodic drills
7. Job descriptions
8. Previous medical records promptly available to Emergency Department staff
9. Protocol for securing cardio-pulmonary bypass for patients for whom it is required
10. 24 hour availability of representative of hospital administration

MINIMUM EMERGENCY SERVICE CRITERIA

I. Emergency Department Characteristics
  A. Access to Hospital-Emergency Department Complex
    1. Identification of and access to hospital (2–5 miles)
      a. Signs posted on streets adjacent to hospital and main streets leading to hospital
      b. Directional signs on hospital property designating Emergency Department entrance
      c. Emergency Department accessible to ground transportation in all types of weather
    2. Access to Emergency Department
      a. Clearly marked entrance
      b. Separate outside entrance
      c. Ground level entrance
      d. Doors to permit easy passage of stretchers, wheelchairs, IV equipment
  B. Staffing
    1. 24-hour staffing by on-call physician
    2. 24-hour Emergency Department nursing staff
    3. Availability of attendants capable of assisting in lifting or otherwise transporting patients from one place to another
  C. Plant Layout
    1. Specifically designated areas
      a. Registration space
      b. Examination and treatment space
      c. Physicians' and nurses' work area

   2. Appropriate Emergency Department illumination
   3. Auxiliary power provisions
D. Equipment
   1. Medications and supplies required for most common emergency problems
   2. Sterile surgical sets
   3. Splints
   4. Thoracic and abdominal paracentesis sets
   5. Intravenous fluids and administration devices
   6. Suction devices
   7. Gastric lavage equipment
   8. Equipment for ventilation
   9. Intubation tray
   10. Tracheostomy tray
   11. Catheterization tray
   12. Wall or portable oxygen
   13. Electrocardiograph
   14. Cardiac monitor-defibrillator
   15. Central venous monitoring setups
   16. Closed thoracostomy tray
   17. Wheelchairs
   18. Stretchers
E. Policies
   1. Written procedures for the procurement of equipment and medications
   2. Open 24 hours a day
   3. Medical records maintained on all patients
   4. Protocol for notification of a patient's family and personal physician as established by hospital staff
   5. Patients accepted for treatment without regard to race, creed, sex, color, or determination of ability to pay
   6. Emergency Department references regarding tetanus, burn, wounds and other emergency problems
   7. Predetermined plan for diagnosis and treatment of the alcoholic or drug abuse patient
   8. Regular audit of records
   9. Continuing Education Program for all Emergency Department Personnel
   10. Maintenance of poison control index and communication with Poison Control Center
   11. System for patient follow-up care as established by hospital medical staff

       12. Communications with other municipal, state and federal health agencies

  F. Communications

    1. Intra-hospital communication by telephone

    2. Communication with ambulance services

II. Characteristics of Hospital Operating an Emergency Department

  A. Backup Medical Staffing

    1. *Promptly available* under normal conditions and circumstances.

      a. Anesthesiologist

      b. Clinician/physician capable in managing surgical and non-surgical emergencies

  B. Backup Non-Physician Manpower

    1. *On call, 24 hours*

      a. Laboratory Staff

      b. Radiologic Staff

      c. Blood bank Staff

      d. Respiratory Therapist

      e. Operating room and delivery staff

  C. Physical Plant

    1. Medical-surgical capability to give at least initial intensive care to all types of patients with emergencies commonly requiring such care

    2. Operating rooms available, 24 hours

    3. Blood bank within the facility (a medical facility within the hospital, staffed by qualified technicians and under the medical direction of a physician capable of and responsible for the procurement, drawing, processing, storage and distribution of whole blood and plasma)

    4. Postoperative recovery area available 24 hours and staffed whenever patients are present

    5. Central sterile supply room

    6. Hospital switchboard—open 24 hours

    7. Admitting Office

    8. Medical records department

    9. Morgue

  D. Support Services Available

    1. Proctoscopy

    2. Bronchoscopy

    3. Radiology (plain and contrast studies)

    4. Laboratory (for indispensable laboratory tests related to emergency medical problems)

     5. Blood bank

     6. Respiratory therapy

E. Policies

     1. Specific definition of administration of Emergency Department

     2. General written policies as guides for Emergency Department personnel

     3. Emergency Department record incorporated into the patient's hospital record if patient is admitted

     4. Admitting office representative available 24 hours

     5. Ready access by Emergency Department to other space, equipment, supplies and drugs

     6. Written Disaster Plan with periodic drills

     7. Job descriptions

     8. Protocol for securing cardio-pulmonary bypass for patients for whom it is required

     9. 24 hour availability of representative of hospital administration

Notes

Notes to Preface
1. Yale Trauma Program, A Proposal to the Commonwealth Fund, 1969.

PART I PERSPECTIVE AND PLANNING

Notes to Chapter 1
EMS in Perspective: The Past Decade
1. "International Trauma Symposium: Research on the Care of the Injured," *Journal of Trauma* 10, 11 (November, 1970): 911–1101.

2. U.S. Department of Health, Education and Welfare, National Center for Health Statistics, Public Health Service Health Resources Administration, *Vital Statistics of the United States* 2 (1973): 441–443.

3. C.F. Frey, D.F. Huelke, and P.W. Gikas, "Resuscitation and Survival in Motor Vehicle Accidents," *Journal of Trauma* 9, 4 (1969): 292–310.

4. S. Cretin, "A Model of the Risk of Death from Myocardial Infarction," Technical Report 09-74, Operations Research Center, Massachusetts Institute of Technology, Cambridge, Mass., 1974.

5. Committee Report, No. 93-397, "Emergency Medical Services Systems Act of 1973," Senate Committee on Labor and Public Welfare, 93rd Congress, 1st Session, September 18, 1973, p. 25. (Hereafter cited as Committee Report.)

6. National Academy of Sciences, National Research Council, Division of Medical Sciences, Report, "Accidental Death and Disability: The Neglected Disease of Modern Society," Washington, D.C., 1966.

7. National Academy of Sciences, National Research Council, Division of Medical Sciences, Committee on Emergency Medical Services, "Roles and Resources of Federal Agencies in Support of Comprehensive Emergency Systems" (Washington, D.C.: National Research Council, March 1972), p. 3. (Hereafter cited as NRC Report.)

8. Ibid., pp. 14-20.

9. Committee Report, p. 26.

10. Hearings Before the Sub-Committee on Public Health and the Environment of the Committee on Interstate and Foreign Commerce, House of Representatives, Appendix A to the *Emergency Medical Services Act of 1972 (Part II)*, Serial No. 92-84, Washington, D.C., June 13-15, 1972. See also: Highway Safety Programs Manual, Vol. 11, "Emergency Medical Services," U.S. Department of Transportation (January 1969).

11. NRC Report, p. 20.

12. Personal communication, Robert Motley, National Highway Traffic Safety Program, Department of Transportation (June 1976).

13. National Academy of Sciences, National Research Council, Division of Medical Services, "Advanced Training for Emergency Medical Technicians-Ambulance," Washington, D.C., September 1970.

14. Personal communication, Robert Motley (June 1976).

15. Hearings Before the Sub-Committee on Public Health and the Environment of the Committee on Interstate and Foreign Commerce, House of Representatives, Military Assistance to Safety and Traffic Program (MAST), "Report of Test Program by the Interagency Study Group," U.S. Department of Defense, Department of Transportation, Department of Health, Education and Welfare (1970), Appendix A to the *Emergency Medical Services Act of 1972 (Part I)*, Serial No. 92-84, Washington, D.C., June 13-15, 1972, pp. 146-150. For additional analyses of the MAST program see M.D. Keller and W.R. Gemma, "A Study of Military Assistance in Safety and Traffic (MAST); San Antonio, Texas," Ohio State University, Department of Preventive Medicine, Columbus, Ohio (July 1971) and Stanford Research Institute, "Evaluation of Operations and Marginal Costs of MAST Alternatives," U.S. Army, Office of the Chief of Staff, Washington, D.C., October 1971.

16. Department of Health, Education and Welfare Report to the Congress, "Emergency Medical Services," in *Hearings on the Emergency Medical Services Systems Act of 1973*, Committee on Interstate and Foreign Commerce, House of Representatives, Washington, D.C., March 15, 1973, p. 99. (Hereafter cited as Hearings.)

17. Department of Health, Education and Welfare, "Report of the Secretary's Advisory Committee on Traffic Safety," Washington, D.C., February 29, 1968, p. xii.

18. Department of Health, Education and Welfare, "Final Report of the Surgeon General's Steering Committee on Emergency Health Care and Injury Control," Washington, D.C., June 1970.

19. Richard Nixon, State of the Union Message, January 20, 1972.

20. Richard Nixon, "President's Message on the Health Care System," House of Representatives Document No. 92-261, Washington, D.C., March 2, 1972, p. 13.

21. Hearings, p. 99.

22. Testimony of Dr. John S. Zapp, deputy assistant secretary for health legislation, Department of Health, Education and Welfare, in *Hearings on the*

Emergency Medical Services Systems Act of 1973, Committee on Interstate and Foreign Commerce, House of Representatives, Washington, D.C., March 15, 1973, p. 72.

23. Public Law 93-641, December 1974.

24. Hearings, Sub-Committee on Public Health and the Environment of the Committee on Interstate and Foreign Commerce, House of Representatives, Washington, D.C., June 13–15, 1972.

25. The Washington, D.C., hearings were held March 15, 1973.

26. The House/Senate Conference report was approved in July 1973.

27. Richard M. Nixon, "Veto Message on Emergency Medical Services Systems Development Act, S-920-7," Washington, D.C., August 2, 1973.

28. Committee Report, p. 21.

29. Committee Report, p. 22.

30. National Emergency Medical Services Information Clearinghouse, Report, "Evaluation of Emergency Medical Services: Basic Guidelines," Department of Community Medicine, University of Pennsylvania, Philadelphia, Pennsylvania, 1975.

31. Bulletin No. 73-1 from Mr. Clay T. Whitehead, director, Office of Telecommunications Policy, executive office of the President, "In Regard to National Policy for Emergency Telephone Number 911," March 21, 1973.

32. IRAC Report, p. 11.

33. Federal Communications Commission, "Medical Communications Services," *Federal Register* 39, 137, Part III (July 16, 1974): 26116–126.

34. HEW Guidelines, p. 15.

35. Personal communication, Dr. John Beck, University of California School of Medicine, San Francisco, July 1976.

36. H. Plaas et al., "The Evaluation of Policy Related Research on Emergency Medical Services," Bureau of Public Administration, University of Tennessee, Knoxville, Tennessee, 4 vols., August 30, 1974.

37. Ibid., Volume IV, pp. 19–22. The need for quality research in EMS was presented by G. Gibson in "Emergency Medical Services Research: Integration or Isolation?" *Health Services Research* 9, 4 (Winter 1974): 255–269.

38. President Gerald Ford, "Informal Remarks on Emergency Medical Services," *Tuesday at the White House* (unpublished) (January 6, 1976).

39. T. Cooper, assistant secretary for health, "Statement on Emergency Medical Services before the Sub-Committee on Health, Committee on Labor and Public Welfare, United States Senate," Washington, D.C., January 23, 1976.

40. Senator Alan Cranston, "Opening Statement," Hearings on Emergency Medical Services Systems Act, January 23, 1976, p. 3.

41. G.J. Ahart, director, Manpower and Welfare Division, U.S. General Accounting Office, "Statement on Emergency Medical Services Systems Act of 1973," before Subcommittee on Health, Committee on Labor and Public Welfare, Washington, D.C., January 23, 1976. For the complete report which reaches the same basic conclusions, see: "Progress, But Problems In Developing Emergency Medical Services Systems," Report to the Congress by the Comptroller General of the United States, July 13, 1976.

42. J.M. Frey, Assistant Director for Legislative Reference, Office of Management and Budget, letter to Senator Harrison A. Williams, Jr., Chairman, Committee on Labor and Public Welfare, U.S. Senate, Washington, D.C., February 12, 1976.

43. Public Law 94-573, the Emergency Medical Services Amendments of 1976, Washington, D.C., October 21, 1976. Committee Report, Number 94-889, "Emergency Medical Services Amendments of 1976," 94th Congress, 2nd Session, May 14, 1976.

Notes to Chapter 2
Launching the Connecticut Study—
Plan and Methodology

1. G. Gibson, "Emergency Medical Services: The Research Gaps," *Health Services Research* 9, 1 (Spring 1974): 6-21; "Guidelines for Research and Evaluation of Emergency Medical Services," *Health Services Reports* 89, 2 (March-April 1974): 99-111. See also: T. Willemain, "The Status of Performance Measures For Emergency Medical Services," *Technical Report No. 06-74*, Massachusetts Institute of Technology (July 1974).

2. G. Gibson, "Evaluation Criteria for Emergency Ambulance Systems," *Social Science and Medicine* 7 (1973): 425-54.

3. It is often assumed that EMS resources—particularly ambulance services—do not meet consumer needs, but recent evidence suggests that "overresponse" can be as much of a problem as "underresponse." K.J. Keggi, S.B. Webb, Jr., and E. Broadbent, "A Methodology for Studying the Emergency Care of the Trauma Patient: Results of the Yale Trauma Study," *Connecticut Medicine* 34, 2 (Feb. 1970): 107-14; S.B. Webb, Jr. and J. Christoforo, "The Use and Misuse of Ambulance Services by the Population Using the Emergency Department at the Hospital of St. Raphael," *Connecticut Medicine* 38, 4 (April 1974): 195-97.

4. "A Study and Analysis of Emergency Medical Services in Connecticut," A Report to the Governor of Connecticut and the Department of Transportation, Vols. 1 and 2, Trauma Program, Department of Surgery, Yale University School of Medicine, December 15, 1972.

5. A.M. Sadler, Jr., B.L. Sadler, and S.B. Webb, Jr., "Emergency Medical Services in Connecticut: A Blueprint for Change," Trauma Program, Department of Surgery, Yale University School of Medicine, New Haven, Connecticut, 1973.

7. Department of Health, Education and Welfare, U.S. Public Health Service, Health Services and Mental Health Association, National Center for Health Services Research and Development, *Uniform Manpower Evaluation Protocol* (Washington, D.C.: U.S. Government Printing Office, April 1971).

PART II THE PRE-HOSPITAL PHASE

Notes to Chapter 3
Emergency Ambulance Services

1. G.J. Curry, "The Immediate Care and Transportation of the Injured," *Bulletin of the American College of Surgeons* 44, 1 (Jan.-Feb. 1959): 32-34, 64-67.

2. "Surgical First Aid Is Available in German City in Ten Minutes," *Hospital Tribune* 3 (July 14, 1969): 14; E. Gogler, "Road Accidents," *Series Chirurgica Geigy* 5 (1962): 78-84; J.F. Pantridge and J.S. Geddes, "A Mobile Intensive Care Unit in the Management of Myocardial Infarction," *The Lancet* 5 (August 5, 1967): 271-73.

3. Whether such mobile coronary-care units are cost-effective, however, is open to question. S. Cretin, "A Model of the Risk of Death from Myocardial Infarction," Technical Report 09-74, Massachusetts Institute of Technology, Operations Research Center, Cambridge, Mass., November 1974.

4. *Roles and Resources of Federal Agencies in Support of Comprehensive Emergency Systems,* Committee on Emergency Medical Services, Division of Medical Services, National Academy of Sciences, National Research Council, Washington, D.C., March 1972, pp. 14-20.

Notes to Chapter 4
Emergency Medical Communications
1. In a 1970 study of the New Haven fire department, nearly 60 percent of all emergency medical assistance (EMA) calls to the fire department ultimately required an emergency ambulance. Paul Browne, "Fire Department Medical Emergency Van Evaluation and System Simulation," master's thesis, Department of Epidemiology and Public Health, School of Medicine, Yale University, New Haven, Connecticut, 1970.

Notes to Chapter 5
Costs of Emergency Ambulance Services
1. These problems have been recognized by others and recently a number of ED cost studies have begun to shed some light on this thorny problem. B.G. King and E.D. Sox, "An Emergency Medical Services System—Analysis of Workload," *Public Health Reports* 82, 11 (November 1967): 995-1008; E.J. Lusk, A.G. Novak, and R.G. Roux, "Emergency Service—How Do You Measure Its Financial Impact?" *Hospital Financial Management* 5, 3 (March 1975): 52-56; R. Leidelmeyer, "The Emergency Department: A Department in Financial Trouble or a Losing Proposition?" *Virginia Medical Monthly* 100 (May 1973): 454-58; G. Bugbee, H. Cook, and W. Mueller, "Emergency Department Losses," *Hospital Financial Management* 25, 10 (Oct. 1971): 3-6; J.D. Thompson and S.B. Webb, Jr., "Effect of the Emergency Department on Hospital Inpatient Services: A Statewide Analysis," *Inquiry* 10, 2 (June 1973): 19-26; K.E. Mangold, "The Financial Realities of Emergency Medical Services," *Hospitals, J.A.H.A.* 47, 10 (May 16, 1973): 89-96; "Evaluation Procedure for Use in the Evaluation of the Financial Impact of Emergency Departments in Hospitals," Report to fulfill the requirements of H.S.M.H.A., Order No. PLD-12164-72 (June 15, 1973).

2. These difficulties are also apparent in the major national study of ambulance costs: Dunlap and Associates, Inc., *The Economics of Highway Emergency Services,* Vols. 1 and 2 (Darien, Conn.: Clearinghouse for Federal Scientific and Technical Information, July 1968). See also: K.J. Keggi, S.B. Webb, Jr., and E. Broadbent, "A Methodology for Studying the Emergency Care of the Trauma

Patient: Results of the Yale Trauma Study," *Connecticut Medicine* 34, 2 (Feb. 1970): 107-14; G. Gibson, *Emergency Medical Services in the Chicago Area* (Chicago: Center for Health Administration Studies, University of Chicago, 1970); B.G. King and E.D. Sox, "An Emergency Medical Service System: Analysis of Workload," *Public Health Reports* 82 (Nov. 1967): 995-1008; E.S. Savas, "Simulation and Cost Effectiveness Analysis of New York's Emergency Ambulance Service," *Management Science* 15, 12 (Aug. 1969): 608-27; K.A. Stevenson, "Emergency Ambulance Service in U.S. Cities: An Overview," *Technical Report No. 40* (Cambridge: Operations Research Center, Massachusetts Institute of Technology, 1968). An analysis of costs and financing of emergency medical services in six selective regional systems has recently been completed by Dr. William Hamilton and associates at the Leonard Davis Institute of the University of Pennsylvania and will soon be published.

3. For a detailed discussion of the effect of monetary subsidies on ambulance service income see Dunlap and Associates, Inc., *The Economics of High-Way Emergency Ambulance Services*, Vols. 1 and 2 (Darien, Connecticut: Clearinghouse for Federal Scientific and Technical Information, July 1968).

4. For a discussion and limited study of this issue see S.B. Webb, Jr., and J. Christoforo, "The Use and Misuse of Ambulance Services by the Population Using the Emergency Department of the Hospital of St. Raphael," *Connecticut Medicine* 38, 4 (April 1974): 195-97.

PART III   THE HOSPITAL PHASE

Notes to Chapter 6
Hospital Emergency Departments

1. The reasons for the increased utilization of hospital emergency departments have been presented by M.L. Webb in "The Emergency Medical Care System in a Metropolitan Area," Ph.D. dissertation, School of Hygiene and Public Health, Department of Medical Care and Hospitals, Johns Hopkins University, 1969; and amplified further by G. Gibson, G. Bugbee, and O. Anderson, *Emergency Medical Services in the Chicago Area* (Chicago: Center for Health Administration Studies, University of Chicago, 1970). The increased rate can be attributed to *population factors* (a 2 percent population growth rate per year, increase in incidence of chronic disease, accident rates, geographically mobile population), *physician factors* (MDs leaving the inner city; unavailability on weekends, holidays, nights; specialization), *hospital factors* (costly equipment for provision of care only available in hospitals, public confidence in hospitals, hospital as only place where care is available twenty-four hours per day), and *external factors* (health insurance plan benefits for emergency department care are available, in contrast to other types of ambulatory care for which no benefits are available; legal issues).

2. R.H. Brook and R.L. Stevenson, Jr., "Effectiveness of Patient Care in an Emergency Room," *New England Journal of Medicine* 283 (October 22, 1970): 904-907.

3. R.M. Sigmond, "Areawide Planning for Emergency Services," *JAMA* 200, 4 (April 24, 1967).

4. P.A. Skudder, J. McCarroll, and P.A. Wade, "Hospital Emergency Facilities and Services: A Survey," *Bulletin of the American College of Surgeons* 46 (March/April 1961): 44-50.

5. P.A. Torrens, and D.G. Yedvab, "Variations Among Emergency Room Populations: A Comparison of Four Hospitals in New York City," *Medical Care* 8, 1 (January-February 1970): 60-75.

6. This figure represents the most recent available statistics from the Connecticut Hospital Association's Outpatient and Emergency Service Activities Report. There were no comparable statistics for one hospital emergency department due to a reorganization. For a discussion and analysis of this issue, see I.P. Boylston, "Resource Use by Emergency Department Ambulances," master's thesis, Yale University School of Medicine, Department of Epidemiology and Public Health, 1975.

7. *Emergency Services: The Hospital Emergency Department in an Emergency Care System* (Chicago, Ill.: American Hospital Association, 1972). *Recommendations of the Conference on the Guidelines for the Categorization of Hospital Emergency Capabilities* (Chicago, Ill.: American Medical Association, 1971). J.J. Hanlon, "Emergency Medical Care as a Comprehensive System," *Health Service Reports* 88, 7 (August/September 1973): 575-587. R.L. Youmans, and A. Brose, "A Basis for Classifying Hospital Emergency Services," *JAMA* 213, 10 (September 7, 1970): 1647-1651. T. Landau, "Considerations of Regionalization and Categorization in Hospital Emergency Planning," master's thesis, Massachusetts Institute of Technology, Cambridge, Mass., February, 1975.

8. B. Smith, "Emergency Department Categorization Inventory Criteria vs. Performance Criteria," Public Technology, Inc., unpublished paper, July 31, 1975.

9. Ibid., p. 20.

10. American Medical Association, *Categorization of Hospital Emergency Capabilities* (Chicago, Ill.: AMA, 1971).

11. Hospital Council of Southern California, *Responsibility to the Community in the Provision of Hospital Emergency Outpatient Services* (Los Angeles, California: The Council, July 1968).

12. D.R. Boyd, "Emergency Medical Services Systems—Program Guidelines," U.S. Department of Health, Education and Welfare, July 1, 1974.

13. S. Cretin, *A Model of the Risk of Death from Myocardial Infarction*, Technical Report 09-74, Operations Research Center, Massachusetts Institute of Technology, Cambridge, Mass., 1974.

14. Connecticut Committee on Trauma, The American College of Surgeons, *A Report Submitted to Director of Emergency Medical Services*, State Department of Health, Connecticut, March 1976.

15. Joint Commission on Accreditation of Hospitals, *Accreditation Manual for Hospitals* (Chicago, Illinois: The Commission, 1970; updated 1973). (Hereafter cited as *Accreditation Manual.*)

16. American Hospital Association, "The Emergency Department in the Hospital: A Guide to Organization and Management," Chicago, Illinois, 1962, p. 35.

17. JCAH, *Accreditation Manual*, p. 72.

18. JCAH, *Accreditation Manual*, p. 71.

19. American College of Surgeons, "Standards for Emergency Departments in Hospitals," reprinted from *Bulletin of the American College of Surgeons* (May-June 1963): 1. (Hereafter cited as "Standards.")

20. JCAH, *Accreditation Manual*, p. 73.

21. Ibid, p. 75.

22. American College of Surgeons, "Standards," p. 2.

23. JCAH, *Accreditation Manual*, p. 75.

24. American Medical Association, *Categorization of Hospital Emergency Capabilities*, p. 7.

25. JCAH, *Accreditation Manual*, p. 75.

26. Ibid, p. 74.

27. American Medical Association, *Categorization of Hospital Emergency Capabilities*, p. 11.

28. H.C. Huntley, "Emergency Health Services for the Nation," *Nebraska State Medical Journal* 55 (December 1970): 736–739. O.P. Hampton, Jr., "Categorization of Hospital Emergency Departments or Hospitals?" *Journal of Trauma* 10, 2 (February 1970). R.L. Youmans and R.A. Brose, "A Basis for Classifying Hospital Emergency Services," *Journal of the American Medical Association* 213, 10 (September 1970): 1647–51.

29. American Medical Association, *Categorization of Hospital Emergency Capabilities*, p. 8.

Notes to Chapter 7
Emergency Department Physicians

1. J.D. Mills, "The Alexandria Plan," *The Emergency Department: A Handbook for Medical Staff* (Chicago: American Medical Association, 1966), p. 17.

2. R.R. Leichtman and M.F. Maravaleas, "The Pontiac Plan," *The Emergency Department: A Handbook for Medical Staff* (Chicago: American Medical Association, 1966), p. 31.

3. The results of the survey performed by the Connecticut Academy of General Practice were furnished by Harry P. Levine, M.D., Stamford, Conn.

4. H. Fenhagen, "The Organization of Physician Manpower in the Emergency Services of the 35 Voluntary General Hospitals in Connecticut," master's thesis, Department of Epidemiology and Public Health, Yale University School of Medicine, New Haven, Connecticut, 1972.

5. Joint Commission on Accreditation of Hospitals, *Accreditation Manual for Hospitals* (Chicago, Illinois: The Commission, 1970; updated 1973), p. 72. The 1970 guidelines of the American College of Surgeons provide that: "Additional members of the medical staff should be on call for consultation and unusual contingencies. The services of specialists should be made available by pre-arrangement." (*Guidelines for Design and Function of a Hospital Emergency Department* [Chicago: The American College of Surgeons, Committee on Trauma, 1970], p. 7).

6. This finding fits with the work of Koughan in his survey of the continuing education of community physicians. W.P. Koughan, "A Description and a Contrast of the Methods by Which Urban and Rural Physicians Obtain Continuing Medical Education," master's thesis, Department of Epidemiology and Public Health, Yale University Medical School, New Haven, Connecticut, 1971. Similarly, the finding is supported in K. Bucholz, "An Appraisal of Genetic Knowledge of Connecticut Pediatricians," master's thesis, Department of Epidemiology and Public Health, Yale University School of Medicine, New Haven, Connecticut, 1976.

Notes to Chapter 8
Emergency Department Nurses and
Other ED Personnel

1. U.S. Department of Health, Education and Welfare, Secretary's Committee Report, "Extending the Scope of Nursing Practice," DHEW Pub. No. 0-720-301 (Washington, D.C.: U.S. Government Printing Office, 1972).

2. The reactions to the basic task list which was provided for physician and nonphysician personnel are not presented here in detail but are available. See G. Starr, "A Description and Analysis of Non-Physician Manpower in Emergency Medical Services in Connecticut," master's thesis, Department of Epidemiology and Public Health, Yale University School of Medicine, New Haven, Connecticut, 1972.

3. For an analysis of issues related to expanding nursing roles and utilization of physician assistants, see A.M. Sadler, Jr., B.L. Sadler, and A.A. Bliss, *The Physician's Assistant: Today and Tomorrow*, 2d ed. (Cambridge, Mass.: Ballinger Publishing Co., 1975).

4. The scheduled man-hours per year provided by the Connecticut Hospital EDs are available for study. See Starr, "Description and Analysis of Non-Physician Manpower," footnote 2.

PART IV   IMPROVING THE SYSTEM

Notes to Chapter 9
Legal and Regulatory Issues

1. For an analysis of other legal issues, see N.L. Chayet, *The Legal Aspects of Emergency Care* (New York: Appleton-Century-Crofts, 1969).

2. *General Statutes of Connecticut*, Vol. V, Revised to 1975, Chapter 370, Section 20-9.

3. E. Forgotson, C. Bradley, and M. Ballenger, "Health Services for the Poor—The Manpower Problem: Innovations and the Law," *Wisconsin Law Review* No. 3 (December 1970): 756–89; A. Leff, "Medical Devices and Paramedical Personnel: A Preliminary Context for Emerging Problems," *Washington University Law Quarterly* 1967, 3 (Summer 1967): 332–413.

4. Council on Health Manpower of the AMA, House of Delegates, *Licensure of Health Occupations* (adopted December 1970); American Hospital Associa-

tion Special Committee on Licensure of Health Personnel, *Statement on Licensure of Health Personnel* (approved November 18, 1970).

5. Department of Health, Education and Welfare, *Report on Licensure and Related Health Personnel Credentialing to the Congress of the United States* (June 1971). For a detailed discussion of these issues, see A.M. Sadler, Jr., B.L. Sadler, and A.A. Bliss, *The Physician's Assistant: Today and Tomorrow*, 2d edition (Cambridge, Mass.: Ballinger Publishing Co., 1975), Chapter 4.

6. B.L. Sadler, J.Q. Tilson, and A.M. Sadler, Jr., "An Analysis of the 1971 Amendment to the Connecticut Medical Practice Act," *Connecticut Medicine* 36, 10 (October 1972): 605-608.

7. N.L. Chayet, *Legal Implications of Emergency Care* (New York: Appleton-Century-Crofts, 1969).

Notes to Chapter 11
Epilogue—1976

1. A.M. Sadler, Jr., B.L. Sadler, and S.B. Webb, Jr., "Emergency Medical Services in Connecticut: A Blueprint for Change," Trauma Program, Department of Surgery, Yale University School of Medicine, New Haven, Connecticut, 1973.

2. "A Study and Analysis of Emergency Medical Services in Connecticut," A Report to the Governor of Connecticut and the Department of Transportation, Vols. 1 and 2, Trauma Program, Department of Surgery, Yale University School of Medicine, December 15, 1972.

3. Sadler, Sadler, and Webb, "Emergency Medical Services in Connecticut," footnote 1.

4. Personal communications with Martin Stillman, J.D., in July 1976.

5. R. Touloukian, M.D., and T.J. Krizek, M.D., *Diagnosis and Early Management of Trauma Emergencies: A Manual for the Emergency Service* (Springfield, Illinois: Charles C. Thomas, 1974).

6. Personal communications with Martin Stillman, J.D., July 1976.

7. R. Brittain, "South Central Connecticut Disaster Planning," master's thesis, Department of Epidemiology and Public Health, Yale University School of Medicine, New Haven, Connecticut, 1974.

8. S.B. Webb, Jr., M.D. Robson, and A. Lanckton, "A Monitoring Strategy for Quality Assurance Programs," *Connecticut Medicine* 39, 4 (April, 1975): 253-256.

9. S.B. Webb, Jr., J.D. Thompson, and I. Whit, "Hospital Resource Use by Emergency and Non-Emergency Diagnostic Specific Admissions," *Inquiry*, 1976 (in press).

10. S.B. Webb, Jr., J.D. Thompson, and I. Whit, "Statewide Trends in Emergency Service Utilization," *Inquiry*, 1976 (in press).

11. E.M. O'Gara, "Categorization of Emergency Services in Connecticut's 35 Short-Term General Hospitals: A Feasibility Study," master's thesis, Department of Epidemiology and Public Health, Yale University School of Medicine, New Haven, Connecticut, 1975.

12. M.C. Robson, *Third Progress Report of the Yale Trauma Program*, Department of Surgery, Yale University School of Medicine, New Haven, Connecticut, 1974.

13. G. Gibson, "Guidelines for Research and Evaluation of Emergency Medical Services," *Health Services Reports* 89, 2 (March–April 1974): 99-110.

14. R.H. Brook and R.L. Stevenson, Jr., "Effectiveness of Patient Care in an Emergency Room," *New England Journal of Medicine* 283 (October 22, 1970): 904-907.

15. M.C. Robson, S.B. Webb, Jr., and A. Lanckton, "Emergency Room Testing of Skull Fracture Patients: Minimum Standards and Performance," *Connecticut Medicine* 39, 5 (May 1975): 290-293.

Index

About the Authors

Alfred M. Sadler, Jr. is completing his residency training in internal medicine at the Massachusetts General Hospital and is a clinical fellow in Medicine at the Harvard Medical School.

Dr. Sadler was Director of the Yale Trauma Program from 1970 to 1973. During that time he was an Assistant Professor of Surgery and Public Health at the Yale University School of Medicine and directed the Yale Physicians' Associate Program. He served as Project Director of the state-wide study of Connecticut emergency medical services and as the first chairman of the Connecticut Advisory Committee on Emergency Medical Services from 1971 to 1973. He co-authored, with Mr. Sadler and Ann A. Bliss, *The Physician's Assistant: Today and Tomorrow.*

From 1973 to 1976, Dr. Sadler was an Assistant Vice President of The Robert Wood Johnson Foundation, Princeton, New Jersey, where he was heavily involved in the development of health manpower and quality of care programs.

During three years at the National Institutes of Health as a commissioned officer in the U.S. Public Health Service from 1967 to 1970 he was engaged in medical-legal and health policy analysis including the preparation and design of the Uniform Anatomical Gift Act which has been enacted in all states. He served as special assistant to Dr. Roger O. Egeberg (Assistant Secretary for Health) for whom he co-authored a report on the licensure and certification of health personnel.

Dr. Sadler is a graduate of Amherst College and Hahnemann Medical School and did postgraduate training in surgery at the Hospital of the University of Pennsylvania. He is a member of Alpha Omega Alpha.

Blair L. Sadler is Assistant Vice President of The Robert Wood Johnson Foundation, Princeton, New Jersey.

Mr. Sadler was an Assistant Professor of Law at Yale University and Co-Director of the Yale Trauma Program from 1970 to 1973. During that period, he served as Counsel to the Yale Physicians' Associate Program.

He served as Co-Project Director of the state-wide study of Connecticut emergency medical services and was a member of the Connecticut Advisory Committee on Emergency Medical Services from 1971 to 1973. He is a member of the National Academy of Sciences Committee on Emergency Medical Services and has served as a consultant to the Department of Health, Education and Welfare in this field. Mr. Sadler has been heavily involved in the development of The Robert Wood Johnson Foundation programs in emergency medical care. He co-authored, with Dr. Sadler and Ann A. Bliss, *The Physician's Assistant: Today and Tomorrow.*

During three years at the National Institutes of Health as a commissioned officer in the U.S. Public Health Service from 1967 to 1970 he was engaged in medical-legal and health policy analysis including the preparation and design of the Uniform Anatomical Gift Act which has been enacted in all states. He served as a special assistant to Dr. Roger O. Egeberg (Assistant Secretary for Health) for whom he co-authored a report on the licensure and certification of health personnel.

Mr. Sadler is a graduate of Amherst College and the University of Pennsylvania Law School, is a member of the Pennsylvania Bar, and served as a Law Clerk for two years with the Superior Court of Pennsylvania.

Samuel B. Webb, Jr. is Associate Professor of Public Health and Director, Program in Hospital Administration at the Yale University School of Medicine, Department of Epidemiology and Public Health. He was one of the original members of the Connecticut State Advisory Committee to the Commissioner of Health on EMS and Secretary-Treasurer of the Connecticut Committee on Trauma, American College of Surgeons. He is a consultant on EMS to the National Center for Health Services Research and Development and the Association of University Programs in Health Administration. Currently his research interests concentrate on various aspects of the organization and costs of EMS within and without the hospital and he is the principal investigator of a large scale project investigating the epidemiology and costs of acute spinal cord injury in Connecticut and its relationship to EMS.

Dr. Webb received his B.A. in American Studies from Yale College in 1961 and his M.P.H. with a major in Hospital Administration from Yale in 1963. He worked at Montefiore Hospital in New York City and as a commissioned officer (Lt. Cmdr.) in the U.S. Public Health Service prior to receiving his doctoral degree in Public Health from the University of California at Los Angeles in 1970. He has been a member of the faculty at the Yale University School of Medicine since 1968. He is a member of Delta Omega and Sigma Xi. This year he is on sabbatical leave as consulting epidemiologist to the Spinal Cord Injuries Unit, Stoke-Mandeville Hospital, Aylesbury, England.